Waardenburg Syndrome

Genetic Syndromes and Communication Disorders Series

Robert J. Shprintzen, Ph.D.
Series Editor

Waardenburg Syndrome by Alice Kahn, Ph.D.

Waardenburg Syndrome

A Volume in the
Genetics and Communication Disorders Series

Alice Kahn, Ph.D.

Department of Speech Pathology and Audiology
Miami University
Oxford, Ohio

With contributions from
Kathleen Hutchinson, Ph.D. and Laura J. Kelly, Ph.D.

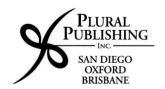

PLURAL
PUBLISHING
INC.

SAN DIEGO
OXFORD
BRISBANE

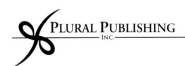

5521 Ruffin Road
San Diego, CA 92123

e-mail: info@pluralpublishing.com
Web site: http://www.pluralpublishing.com

49 Bath Street
Abingdon, Oxfordshire OX14 1EA
United Kingdom

Typeset in 11/13 Garamond by Flanagan's Publishing Services, Inc.
Printed in the Hong Kong by Paramount Printing

For permission to use material from this text, contact us by
Telephone: (866) 758-7251
Fax: (888) 758-7255
e-mail: permissions@pluralpublishing.com

ISBN-13: 978-1-59756-021-4
ISBN-10: 1-59756-021-9

Library of Congress Cataloging-in-Publication Data

Kahn, Alice, 1946-
   Waardenburg syndrome / Alice Kahn.
      p. ; cm. – (Genetic syndromes and communication disorders series)
   Includes bibliographical references and index.
   ISBN-13: 978-1-59756-021-4 (softcover)
   ISBN-10: 1-59756-021-9 (softcover)
   1. Deafness–Genetic aspects. I. Title. II. Series.
   [DNLM: 1. Hearing Loss–genetics. 2. Waardenburg's Syndrome–diagnosis.
   3. Waardenburg's Syndrome–therapy. WV 270 K12w 2006]
   RF292.K34 2006
   617.8'042–dc22
                                       2006015200

Contents

Foreword

*I*t is possible that we are living in a time where more discoveries and technologic advances have been made than at any other time in human history. I can relate this to my own personal life as I reach my 60th birthday this year. I remember as a child, just after World War II, sitting in the living room with my family around a large console radio listening to *The Shadow*, *Fibber McGee and Molly*, and the *Inner Sanctum*. The first television in our house in the early 1950s seemed so unbelievable with three entire channels to watch. The excitement when I was in sixth grade was the race between the Soviets and Americans to put the first satellite in orbit and, later, the first man in space. Color television followed, although only one person in our neighborhood had a color set that received the single television show that was broadcast in color. Then the first jet airliner that reduced the flying time between New York and Miami from over four hours to under two. The wonder of 8-track tape players in cars in the 1960s, and BetaMax videotape recorders at home in the 1970s. I recall the first computer I bought for my office in the early 1980s for over $5,000. Imagine the excitement over a computer with 64 kilobytes of memory and dual 8-inch floppy disk drives. And now, here we are in a new century with gigantic digital televisions, DVD recorders, MP3 players, 200 channels of television delivered by satellite, and the computer I am typing this document on that has more capabilities than computers that occupied an entire room 30 years ago and even then, they only stored data on tape or punch cards. What a time to be living in.

As amazing as our day-to-day lives are compared to 50 years ago, the same is true of the world of science, especially the study of human disease. I remember my first course in genetics in 1967 during my senior year in college. That class followed by just a bit more than a decade the discovery in 1956 that humans actually had 46 chromosomes and not 48 like gorillas and chimpanzees. Only three years before that discovery, Watson and Crick described the double helix structure of DNA in 1953 for which they would win the Nobel prize. In 1967, we studied *Drosophila melanogaster* (fruit flies) to understand inheritance patterns and a limited number of abnormalities caused by presumed mutations in their genes, none of which we could confirm scientifically. Techniques for molecular genetic analysis had not yet been developed. DNA sequencing was developed in 1972 by Sanger, a development that allowed the study of the genetic code in much greater detail. Clinically, the science of clinical genetics began to evolve in the 1970s and 1980s with a spate of newly recognized genetic diseases being described. In the 1990s, as molecular genetics techniques began to become commonplace, the causes of many of these disorders discovered by clinicians became common. More importantly, as the genetic code was cracked, the manner in which genes caused specific diseases was uncovered. The Human Genome Project was begun in October of 1990. The goal of the multinational study was to completely sequence the human genome and to identify all human genes. Originally slated to last for 15 years, the Human Genome Project was completed two years early, almost exactly 50 years after Watson and Crick's discovery. Along the way, the science of "genetics" became relabeled "genomics" and the field of "proteomics" was born to trace how the proteins for which genes encode make traits occur. Few people would argue that this burst of rapid progress in the field of genomics is the most important advancement in the field of human biology in recorded history.

The purpose of the previous two paragraphs was not to provide a parallel trip down memory lane. Putting the most important advancement in health care in the perspective of modern history was necessary in order to ask ourselves, "Am I a part of this history?" In our fields of study, such as speech pathology, audiology, psychology, learning disabilities, child development, and related fields, are we familiar with these advances? Do we understand them? Do we recognize genetic disorders in people we treat? Is it important for us to understand genomics? Are we going to be simple observers in this burst of progress, or participants? These questions are, of course, rhetorical. As Goethe said in the 18th century, "Nature knows no pause in progress and development and attaches her curse on all inaction." Clinicians and scientists who do not understand how genomic variation results in hearing loss, speech problems, educational challenges, and developmental disorders run the risk of being rendered obsolete. There is substantial and strong evidence that speech, language, hearing, cognitive, behavioral, and developmental disorders are often (if not the majority of the time) caused by factors that can be traced back to the genome. Having genomic evidence will lead to more effective predictions of prognosis and treatment, and may even lead to treatments that have not yet been devised. It is possible that our entire approach to communicative and developmental disorders may need to be overhauled once we understand all of the links between genomics and human behavior.

This volume represents the first in a larger series to follow on genomic disorders and how they affect human behavior, communication, development, and treatment. Plural Publishing has identified a vacuum in this field that requires filling, and we will attempt to bring to light a broad range of topics that break down the barriers between the molecular science of genomics and the clinical fields that focus on rehabilitation of speech, hearing, behavioral, and cognitive disorders. The authors represented in this series, including Dr. Kahn and her colleagues who have brought you this volume, represent forward thinkers who have recognized the need to propel the behavioral sciences into the 21st century alongside the rest of human health care. This is an important contribution and the volumes that will follow will form a core of cutting edge material that will prove invaluable to clinicians in practice today.

Robert J. Shprintzen, Ph.D.
Series Editor

Preface

A student once asked me if there were genetic syndromes that had only positive characteristics. For example, could there be a syndrome with a phenotype of blond hair, blue eyes, straight nose, orthognathic profile, and tall stature? Or, stated another way, do families who have very physically attractive, physically and mentally normal family members have a "good" syndrome that can be inherited in the way that "bad" syndromes can be inherited? These questions led to an intriguing discussion and to the conclusion that there are no "good" genetic syndromes because, by definition, "syndrome" means an aggregate of symptoms or signs associated with a disease process or genetic disorder.

The student's question emphasized the commonly held assumption that all syndromes produce unattractive physical features and that persons with genetic syndromes must, by definition, be unattractive. At the very least, such persons must differ so markedly from the accepted social standards of "normal" that they attract unfavorable attention from society as a whole. In general this assumption is accurate, although the definition of "attractive" varies among racial and ethnic groups and by current media depictions of what constitutes fashionable attractiveness. The method of recognizing syndromic phenotypes based on *unattractive* physical features has two important diagnostic implications. First, if an individual who has a genetic syndrome is also physically attractive, he or she is less likely to be diagnosed as "syndromic" and in need of treatment. Second, if the most severe signs of the syndrome are invisible (as is hearing loss), he or she is unlikely to be correctly diagnosed at all.

Waardenburg syndrome is a genetic syndrome that can produce moderate to profound sensorineural hearing loss, as well as distinctive eye, hair, and skin color, and unusual facial features. It differs from other genetic syndromes because the majority of phenotypic features can be concealed, and because some of the phenotypic features such as bright blue eyes are considered physically attractive. Other features, such as a white forelock, are regarded as unusual, but not unattractive, and many people with normal hair color bleach their hair to obtain such a streak. Finally, family members are often unaware that their facial appearance and their hearing loss are part of the same condition. Variability of phenotypic expression may produce attractive looking family members with or without hearing loss; unusual looking family members with or without hearing loss; and/or very unusual looking family members with or without hearing loss. It takes a trained observer to reveal the relationship between hearing loss and facial appearance in Waardenburg syndrome.

This book is designed to present the reader with basic information about the genetic syndrome called Waardenburg (WS) in all its forms. It begins by defining basic genetic concepts and continues by describing the major and minor phenotypic features of four types of WS. This text describes a plan for identifying, diagnosing, and treating patients with WS, incorporates suggestions for counseling families who have the gene for WS, and presents resources for appropriate referral and treatment for WS patients.

Because the phenotype of WS resembles several other genetic and physical conditions such as albinism, piebaldism, and vitiligo, these conditions are summarized and compared to WS. After reading this textbook you should be able to:

- Define and distinguish between WS types 1, 2, 3, and 4.

- Identify the major and minor phenotypic features that may indicate the presence of any type of WS.

- Select the specific types of communication disorders that accompany WS.

- List the types of hearing losses that are associated with WS.

- Recognize the pure tone audiogram patterns that often accompany hearing losses caused by WS.

- Compile a recommended plan of action for treating and referring individuals with WS.

- Understand your role as a health care professional in recognizing, treating, and referring individuals with WS.

- Explain the need for team management in treating individuals with WS, and know where to locate professional craniofacial teams.

- List three syndromes that are similar to WS, and distinguish between the phenotypic features of those syndromes and the phenotypic features of WS.

- Summarize the continuing needs and unanswered questions related to diagnosis and treatment of individuals with WS.

- List specific resource organizations that treat patients with WS.

Contributors

Kathleen Hutchinson, Ph.D.
Professor and Chair, Department of Speech Pathology and Audiology
Miami University of Ohio.

Dr. Hutchinson is currently investigating sensory deprivation among deaf children, the effects of exercise, fitness and muscle strength on hearing ability, and audiologic management of geriatric and preschool populations.

Dr. Laura Kelly, Ph.D., CCC-A
Associate Professor Audiology
Miami University of Ohio

Dr. Kelly teaches courses in amplification, hearing loss management, and electronystagmography (ENG). Her research interests include counseling, attitudes toward hearing impairment and the perception of speech by individuals with normal hearing and hearing loss.

Acknowledgments

We wish to acknowledge Amy Locaputo, B.S., who completed her degree in speech pathology and audiology at Miami University. Her assistance and generosity were greatly appreciated in the compilation of chapter 5. Our thanks to Jennifer Whaley, M.A., speech pathology, at Miami University for her assistance in constructing a WS family support Web site and to Jamie Pratzel, B.S., audiology and speech pathology at Miami University, for her highly professional photographic and content contributions to the Web site, and to chapter 2.

We also wish to thank the individuals who have Waardenburg syndrome, and their families, for allowing us to use their photographs, interview materials, and case histories in this textbook.

We appreciate the assistance of Kathleen Arnos, Ph.D., Director, Genetics Program, Department of Biology, Gallaudet University and Dr. Colleen Jackson-Cook, Cytogenetics Diagnostic Laboratory, Department of Pathology, Virginia Commonwealth University for providing the photograph of a human male karyotype.

This book is dedicated to Dr. G. A. McCarty, Jr. and Dr. Joel Kahane.

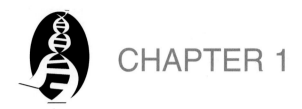

CHAPTER 1

Introduction: Basic Concepts

As a result of the Human Genome Project, the entire human genetic code has been sequenced. Research efforts are now turning to identification of mutations in single genes that cause syndromes. As more information about syndromes becomes available, there is increasing need for health care practitioners to acquire or update their knowledge of basic genetics and to apply this knowledge in diagnosis and treatment of their patients. I have often heard speech-language pathologists and audiologists express the opinion that syndrome identification "is a genetic counselor's job," and that time constraints and professional demands prevent them from recognizing and referring patients who are at risk for genetic disorders. It is true that laboratory analysis, interpretation of DNA testing, and genetic counseling are geneticists' responsibilities. However, someone must initially identify the need for a geneticist's expertise. This means that all health care professionals must acquire and continually update their knowledge of current genetic information. Failure to do so has long-term diagnostic, treatment, and ethical implications for our patients.

Differential diagnostics is a part of every clinician's responsibilities, and in no area is this more important than in the diagnosis and treatment of hearing loss. Hearing loss results from a wide variety of causes, including viral illnesses, head trauma, neoplasms, noise exposure, and hereditary factors. The diagnosis, prognosis, and treatment plans for each type of hearing loss have a different impact on the individual and his or her family members. Syndrome-based hearing losses, including hearing loss from Waardenburg syndrome (WS), are unique and require special training to recognize, diagnose, and treat.

Differential diagnosis of genetic syndromes is a daunting task because thousands of syndromes have been identified. Syndromes with hearing loss as a component are almost as numerous. Toriello, Reardon, and Gorlin (2004) alone describe more than 500 syndromes with hereditary hearing loss as a feature. Health care professionals who diagnose and treat hearing loss must acquire a background of basic genetic knowledge, and keep that background current, if they are to provide the best services to their clients. One of the most compelling reasons for diagnosing syndrome-related hearing loss is that the hereditary hearing losses impact not only the initial patient, but generations of individuals. Failure to recognize and refer someone who has a syndrome affects the treatment outcome not only of the individual seeking treatment, but the individual's family members as well.

Individuals with syndromes have special treatment needs, including genetic testing and genetic counseling. This means that all health care professionals must develop a heightened awareness of what syndromes are and how to recognize and diagnose them. They should also understand the etiology, natural history, and prognosis of the syndromes they are most likely to encounter. After reading this chapter you should be able to:

- Explain what a *genetic* syndrome is.

- List three ways scientists diagnose WS.

- Explain the difference between WS *phenotype* and WS *genotype.*

- List the uses of a family *pedigree* in diagnosing and treating WS.

- Define and explain the difference between the *etiology, natural history,* and *prognosis* for WS.

- Describe how WS was first recognized and named.

- Compare *autosomal dominant* and *autosomal recessive* inheritance patterns.

SYNDROMES

The general term *syndrome* means an aggregate of symptoms or signs associated with a disease process or genetic disorder. Syndromes may originate in a variety of ways. Carpal tunnel syndrome, for example, results from entrapment of the median nerve at the wrist, within the carpal tunnel. Individuals who are employed in situations requiring repetitive movement of the wrist and fingers may develop carpal tunnel syndrome over time. This type of syndrome is not inherited. Horner syndrome describes an abnormal reaction of the pupil of the eye on exposure to light. The abnormal response may result from neoplasms, trauma, or brainstem injury, and is not necessarily a birth anomaly.

Genetic syndromes may result from changes in chromosomes or, in the case of WS, from changes in genes located on chromosomes. In general, genetic factors are believed to cause about one-third of all birth defects, and nearly 85% of congenital anomalies with known causes (Moore & Persaud, 2003). Individuals with genetic syndromes such as WS usually have one or more physical anomalies, all of which originate from a single cause (Jorde, Carey, Bamshad, & White, 2006). All human cells, except for egg and sperm cells, normally have 23 chromosomes. Each chromosome contains genes, which consist of deoxyribonucleic acid (DNA). To identify a syndrome, scientists study an individual's chromosomes, DNA sequence, physical appearance, and family background. Specific identification techniques include karyotyping, genotyping, phenotyping, and pedigree construction.

KARYOTYPE

Karyotyping was developed in the 1950s, and is still used if chromosome rearrangements are suspected. A *karyotype* is a display of an individual's chromosomes, arranged in a specific order. The process begins by having an individual submit a blood or tissue sample for laboratory analysis. After the tissue sample is cultured and chemically treated, the chromosomes are photographed and the photographic pairs of chromosomes are arranged in order according to length and banding characteristics. The patient's chromosomes are then assessed in relation to the well-documented structure of normal chromosomes. Figure 1–1 shows the karyotype of a normal male individual. Abnormal chromosomes may differ from normal ones in several ways: extra chromosomes may be present; all, or part, of the chromosome may be missing; or parts of one chromosome may be broken off and transposed onto another chromosome. Chromosomal additions, deletions, and transpositions produce recognizable syndromes. Because chromosomes each contain hundreds of individual genes, chromosomal anomalies often produce very serious, even lethal effects. Chromosomal syndromes with associated hearing loss include Down syndrome (trisomy 21) and Klinefelter syndrome. Waardenburg syndrome (WS) is *genetic* in etiology and not caused by chromosomal rearrangement. It cannot be detected by karyotyping because genetic syndromes are caused by mutations in genetic material too small to be seen with a microscope. Health care professionals must use other means to diagnose individuals with WS, including phenotyping, genotyping, and preparation of a family pedigree.

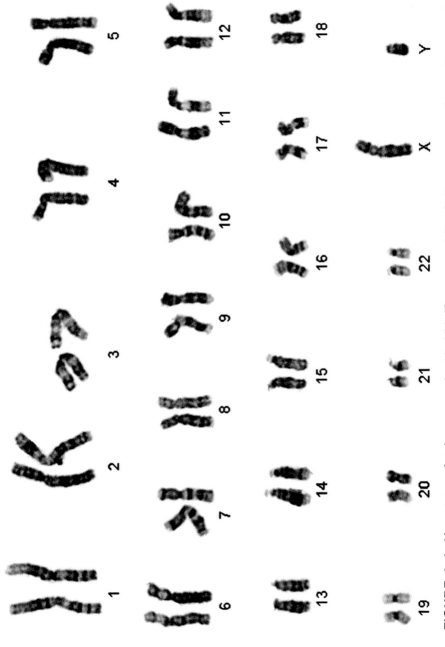

FIGURE 1–1. Karyotype of a human male 46, XY. (Courtesy of Dr. Colleen Jackson-Cook, Cytogenetics Diagnostic Laboratory, Department of Pathology, Virginia Commonwealth University.)

PHENOTYPE

Phenotypic characteristics are those that can be quantified or described in some way. Phenotypes include physical characteristics as well as behavioral ones. The phenotype of someone with Waardenburg syndrome type 1 (WS 1, for example, includes bright blue eyes, heterochromia, sensorineural hearing loss, dystopia canthorum, and normal cognition.

Phenotypes alone are not a certain way to diagnose syndromes because some syndromes have phenotypes that resemble those of other syndromes. It is also possible for an individual to have two or more syndromes, simultaneously displaying phenotypic features of both syndromes. Fortunately, the phenotype of WS is distinctive and geneticists are usually able to readily distinguish it from those of similar syndromes. In some cases, it may still be impossible to determine what, if any, genetic problem the individual has, even after the individual's genotype, phenotype, and pedigree have been examined.

GENOTYPE

A *genotype* is an individual's genetic makeup; it describes the location and type of specific genes located on specific chromosomes. To date, the majority of human genes have been mapped and the entire human genetic code has been sequenced. Using a system of standard nomenclature, scientists can describe the appearance of chromosomes and the exact location of individual genes. Mutations in single genes that cause syndromes are being identified at a rapid rate, and genetic testing for many syndromes is becoming available. Specific tests include DNA mapping, fluorescence in situ hybridization (FISH) testing, and prenatal testing. Such testing is often expensive or experimental, and the costs are often not reimbursed by third-party payers. Waardenburg syndrome has several subtypes, some of which could be detected by genetic testing at the time this book went to press. The locations and nature of mutations causing some WS subtypes have been characterized and are discussed in chapters 2 and 3. Readers who want to acquire in-depth understanding of DNA analysis, FISH testing, the Human Genome Project, or causes of human birth anomalies in general should refer to texts such as those of Cremers and Smith (2002), Jones (1997), Moore and Persaud (2003), and Toriello, Reardon, and Gorlin (2004).

Individuals sometimes want to know why genotyping is needed if they have a phenotype strongly suggestive of WS. Genotyping is needed for several reasons. First, it is the only absolutely certain way to differentially diagnose WS from similar syndromes and medical conditions. These conditions are discussed in detail in chapter 4.

Genotyping is also the only accurate way to distinguish between the various subtypes of WS. Knowing the specific subtype of WS helps clinicians counsel patients about prognosis of hearing loss and health care issues because the inheritance pattern of WS differs among subtypes. For example, WS type 1 has an autosomal dominant transmission pattern, whereas WS type 2 is sometimes autosomal recessive. People with WS often want to know the reproductive risks associated with WS. Knowing the type of inheritance pattern, coupled with preparation of a family pedigree, can help accurately address this issue.

FAMILY PEDIGREE

A *pedigree* is a chart, similar to a genealogy chart. Standard symbols are used to represent family members, and to show those who are affected with a particular disorder. Pedigrees are useful in assisting genetic counselors to decide what inheritance patterns are present in the family, to predict the likelihood of recurrence of a problem in future generations, and to help family members visualize the overall presence of a specific genetic problem within their family. Several types of inheritance patterns exist and each produces a different type of pedigree. For example, autosomal dominant inheritance usually appears as a vertical pattern of genetic transmission, with male and female individuals being equally affected by the disorder (Figure 1-2A). Autosomal recessive inheritance may show a pattern of affected siblings, but no evidence of the disorder in parents (Figure 1-2B). Pedigrees may provide insufficient evidence for diagnosing a particular disorder. The results from pedigree observations are most useful when combined with laboratory findings and a detailed phenotypic analysis. Individuals with genetic syndromes usually want to know not only the recurrence risk of the syndrome, but the etiology of the syndrome and what the effects of the syndrome will be throughout their lifetime.

ETIOLOGY

An *etiology* is a cause of a problem. Fetal alcohol syndrome, for example, occurs because a pregnant woman ingests levels of alcohol sufficient to cause anomalies. Alcohol harms the developing fetus and causes the child to be born with a set of physical and behavioral problems that have been identified as fetal alcohol syndrome. The etiology of many syndromes is known; others are still being delineated. It is clear that continued progress in human genetics will elucidate the causes of most or all genetic diseases in the future.

Key

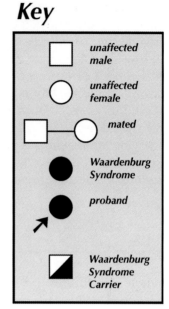

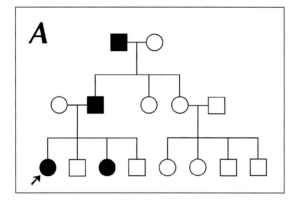

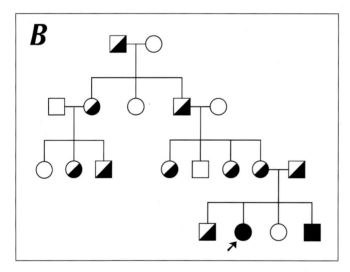

FIGURE 1–2. A. A pedigree representing autosomal dominant inheritance pattern. **B.** A pedigree representing autosomal recessive inheritance pattern.

NATURAL HISTORY

Individuals born with a syndrome are often born with a set of physical problems, some of which may change over the course of the individual's lifetime. Heart disease, diabetes, and mental illness are just a few of the conditions that may occur in individuals with syndromes. Persons who have Marfan syndrome, for example, are usually born with anomalies of the arteries and heart valves, predisposing individuals to heart disease. Individuals with WS have an increased risk of having or developing sensorineural hearing losses during their lifetimes; children with Down syndrome are likely to develop Alzheimer's disease as they age. The likelihood of individuals with a particular syndrome developing problems over time that are associated with that syndrome is called a *natural history*. Not all individuals with WS, for example, will develop hearing loss, but they are at increased risk of doing so. By studying an individual's natural history, health care workers can be prepared for future problems related to hearing loss and communications skills or for an individual's developing a life-threatening condition.

PROGNOSIS

When a health care professional predicts the outcome of an illness or condition, that health care professional is providing the patient with a prognosis. A *prognosis* is a long-term view of the outcome of a situation. A prognosis differs from natural history because it attempts to predict the impact of a condition, the degree of the condition, or the effect that condition will have on the individual's ability to live and function normally. For some lethal or near lethal syndromes the prognosis may be very simple: the child will probably not live longer than 6 months. For syndromes with normal life expectancy, the prognosis often attempts to predict degree of hearing loss, need for surgery or prosthetic management, or special educational needs. For an individual with Waardenburg syndrome (WS), the *natural history* includes development of hearing loss, premature graying of hair, and possibly communication problems resulting from hearing loss. A *prognosis* for that individual might be something like this: if/when a profound hearing loss occurs, this particular child may be a good candidate for a cochlear implant, and she will need aural rehabilitation to learn to communicate with both deaf and normal hearing peers.

A prognosis takes into account factors not directly related to the initial problem (WS). These factors may include general health of the child, economic standing, family support, availability of adequate specialized medical care, and similar matters. Treatment options are formulated based on natural history and prognosis. The earlier a problem is identified, the sooner a prognosis can be made, leading to more effective long-term treatment. For example, because children born with WS are at increased risk of having or developing sensorineural hearing loss, early identification can lead to implementation of prelingual amplification or auditory training to facilitate normal language development. Infant screening programs that use auditory brainstem response (ABR) and otoacoustic emissions testing (OAEs) are one method of early identification for children with cochlear problems, including children with WS. Specific early identification techniques for hearing losses are described in detail in chapter 5.

HISTORY OF WAARDENBURG SYNDROME

P. J. Waardenburg, a Dutch ophthalmologist, initially described the syndrome in 1951. Waardenburg (1951) noticed that many of his patients had anomalies of the eyebrows, nasal root, iris, and scalp and facial hair. He observed that many of these patients were also deaf. Since Waardenburg first published his original description of the syndrome, four distinct types of WS have been identified.

WS is a genetic syndrome with a well-defined phenotype, prognosis, and natural history. It is also an interesting syndrome because a similar genetic condition is found in animals (see shaded box on next page). Research using animal models has demonstrated that the presence of melanocytes is necessary to the normal development of the cochlea and organ of Corti, although the reasons for this are unclear (Steel & Bock, 1983). Pigment-producing cells called melanocytes are normally present in the stria vascularis of the human cochlea. Researchers have speculated that abnormal migration of melanocytes may be responsible for hearing loss in individuals with WS (Toriello, Reardon, & Gorlin, 2004). The human genotypes for some types of WS have been identified. Along with hearing loss, WS produces facial anomalies, and abnormal presence and distribution of pigment to the skin, hair, eyes, and stria vascularis.

Etiology

The genetic mutations that produce WS result from changes in a group of genes called *homeobox* genes. Homeobox genes are responsible for early embryonic development and spatial arrangement of body parts (Moore & Persaud, 2003). Homeobox genes also affect the formation and distribution of pigment-producing cells called melanocytes. *Melanocytes* produce pigment (melanin) that provides skin, eye, and hair color. Melanin is also found in the stria vascularis of the cochlea. Absence of melanin can produce depigmented areas of skin, hair or eyes, and sensorineural hearing loss. Several specific mutations of homeobox genes have been identified. These are discussed in chapters 2 and 3.

Transmission Pattern and Occurrence Rate

Most types of WS have an *autosomal dominant transmission pattern*. This means that there is a 50% chance that a child born to a normal parent and a WS parent will have WS. WS type 4, however, has both autosomal dominant and *autosomal recessive forms*. Individuals with the autosomal recessive form of WS have received a recessive copy of the gene for WS type 4 from both parents. In addition, de novo mutations for all types of WS are possible. In such cases, children may be born to parents who do not have WS. WS occurs in all races and in males and females equally.

WS-Type Problems in Animals

Cat breeders know that white cats with blue eyes, or white cats with odd eyes (one blue eye, one eye of another color) are likely to be deaf (Figure 1–3). If the cat is an odd-eyed cat, the hearing loss is likely to be on the side of the blue eye. This condition is similar to WS in humans, and also occurs in dogs, horses, and the splotch mouse. Deaf cats and dogs make good pets, and can function well in a protected environment, but should never be allowed to run free. Many people mistakenly believe that deaf animals should be destroyed. The Deaf Dogs Web site provides information about the relationship between albinism and hearing loss in dogs and lists deaf dogs that are available for adoption. For more information about deafness in dogs visit http://www.deafdogs.org.

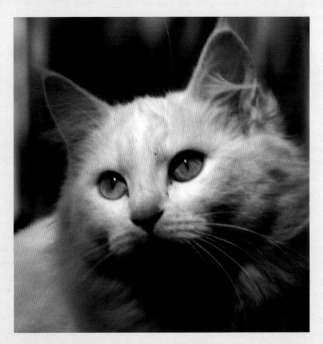

FIGURE 1–3. White cats with blue eyes, or white cats with odd eyes, like this cat, are usually deaf.

The exact incidence of WS is difficult to calculate because incidence reports are often based on specific populations or ethnic groups. Waardenburg originally estimated that 1 in 42,000 individuals in the general population had WS (Newton, 2002). Schaefer (1995), and Read and Newton (1997) estimate that WS occurs in about 1 per 4000 live births, and 1 in 10,000 to 20,000 in the general population, respectively.

The general manifestations of WS appear in most types of the syndrome, but there is phenotypic variability among types. Figure 1–4 demonstrates this variability in four individuals with WS types 1, 2, and 3. Apparently the genetic mutations that produce each type are also distinctly different from one another. We will compare the four types of WS in detail in the following chapters.

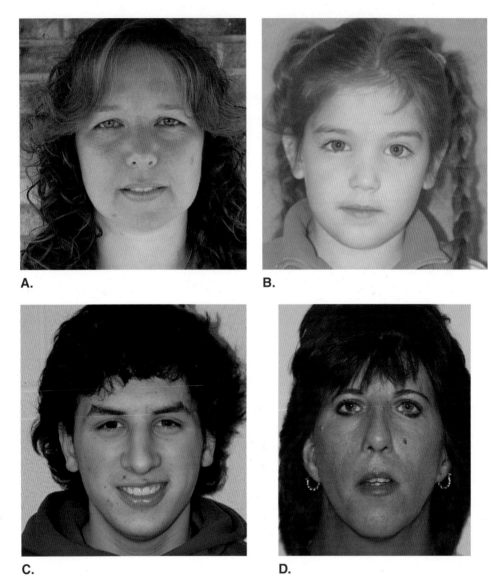

A.   **B.**

C.   **D.**

FIGURE 1–4. The individuals in these photographs show the variability of expression possible for patients with WS. **A.** A young woman who probably has WS1 with heterochromia; **B.** A child with WS1 with normal hearing, bright-blue eyes, hypoplastic nasal alae, and flared eyebrows. **C.** A young man who has WS2, heterochromia, and a profound unilateral hearing loss. **D.** A woman with WS3, synophrys, musculoskeletal anomalies, multiple nevi, heterochromia iridis, and unilateral sensorineural hearing loss.

SUMMARY

In this chapter you have learned:

- What a *genetic syndrome* is.

- The basic methods used to diagnose genetic syndromes.

- The difference between *genotype* and *phenotype*.

- What a pedigree is.

- The difference between etiology, natural history, and prognosis.

- How Waardenburg syndrome was first recognized and named.

REFERENCES

Jones, K. L. (1997). *Smith's recognizable patterns of human malformation* (5th ed.). Philadelphia: W. B. Saunders Co.

Jorde, L., Carey, J., Bamshad, M., & White, R. (2006) *Medical genetics* (3rd ed.). St. Louis: Mosby.

Moore, K. L., & Persaud, T. V. N. (2003). *The developing human. Clinically oriented embryology.* Philadelphia: W. B. Saunders Co.

Newton, V. E. (2002). Clinical features of the Waardenburg syndrome. In Cor W. R. J. Cremers & J. H. Smith (Vol. Eds.), *Advances in oto-rhino-laryngology: Vol. 61. Genetic hearing impairment: Its clinical manifestations* (pp. 201–208). Basel: Karger.

Read, A., & Newton, V. (1997). Waardenburg syndrome. *Journal of Medical Genetics, 34,* 656–665.

Schaefer, B. B. (1995). Ten syndromes most commonly associated with hearing impairment. http://www.boystownhospital.org. Retrieved July 11, 2001.

Steel K. P., & Bock, G. R. (1983). Hereditary inner-ear abnormalities in animals. *Archives of Otolaryngology, 109,* 22–29.

Toriello, H. V., Reardon, W., & Gorlin, R. J. (Eds.). (2004). *Hereditary hearing loss and its syndromes.* Oxford: Oxford University Press.

Waardenburg, P. J. (1951). A new syndrome combining developmental anomalies of the eyelids, eyebrows and nose root with pigmentary defects of the iris and head hair and with congenital deafness. *American Journal of Human Genetics, 3,* 195–253.

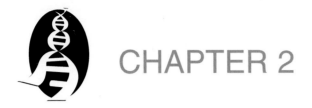

CHAPTER 2

Waardenburg Syndrome Types 1 and 3

*W*aardenburg syndrome is one of more than 400 forms of syndromic deafness, and has been extensively documented since the syndrome was identified in 1951. Until the advent of accurate genetic testing and identification of the WS genes, phenotypic descriptions of patients and pedigree analysis was used to diagnose WS. Genetic testing is now considered the most accurate diagnostic method, but it is not yet available for all types of the syndrome, and it is expensive. Phenotypic descriptions of patients remain a viable method for preliminary identification and differential diagnosis of WS. Four specific types of WS have been identified based on phenotypic descriptions. Because WS type 1 and WS type 3 are phenotypically similar, they are discussed together. This chapter summarizes and compares the phenotypes associated with WS types 1 and 3, and gives suggestions for clinical application of this information to diagnosis and referral of patients with WS. After reading this chapter you should be able to:

- Identify six major phenotypic characteristics of WS type 1.

- List three minor phenotypic characteristics of WS type 1.

- Describe the type of hearing loss that accompanies WS types 1 and 3.

- Name the type of inheritance patterns of WS types 1 and 3.

- Identify the phenotypic characteristics of WS type 3.

- Define *heterochromia iridis* and *dystopia canthorum*.

- Explain the use of the "W Index" in distinguishing WS types 1 and 3 from other types of WS .

13

DIFFERENTIAL DIAGNOSIS OF WS 1 AND WS 3

As health care professionals, we are accustomed to physically observing the individuals in our care. Often this is an informal process focusing on the specifics of our discipline. For example, an ophthalmologist performing a visual examination may observe that her client has bright blue eyes and a white streak of hair in his forehead. If the person's visual skills test out normally, the physician may consider the individual's physical appearance to be interesting, but diagnostically insignificant. In this instance, the physician is correct about the client's visual skills as the individual's appearance is nondiagnostic for *vision* problems. However, by not recognizing the syndromic significance of the patient's appearance, and the broader consequences of that appearance, the physician has failed to provide a complete and accurate assessment of the patient's condition. Individuals with WS, and their relatives, are at increased risk for medical conditions including sensorineural hearing loss, melanoma, cleft palate, spina bifida, and communication disorders secondary to hearing loss. Unless we, as health care professionals, increase our awareness of genetic syndromes and their effects, we risk, at least, being ineffective clinicians and, at worst, harming our patients by not informing them of genetic implications of their condition. To diagnose, refer, and treat individuals with WS, we must recognize the phenotypic features of the syndrome.

The WS phenotype results from genetic errors that, among other things, affect the production and distribution of pigment-producing cells (melanocytes) to the skin, hair, eyes, and inner ear. Pigment (melanin) is the substance that gives color to the iris of the eye, hair, and skin. Moles, or nevi, are also collections of pigment and may be widely distributed on the skin of individuals with WS. The molecular genetics of WS is a topic beyond the scope of this book. Readers who want to acquire a detailed understanding of the molecular basis for WS phenotypes can find it in Toriello, Reardon, and Gorlin's (2004) excellent atlas of hereditary hearing loss syndromes. For most of us, it is sufficient to understand that, when pigment anomalies are present in individuals, those anomalies may indicate the presence of an invisible phenotypic feature: hearing loss.

The phenotypic features of WS have been documented since the mid-1950s, and have been grouped into major and minor categories, with major features occurring frequently, and minor features less so. The *number* of features present in a given individual is significant to differential diagnosis of WS. A person is considered to have WS type 1, for example, if he or she has two major, or one major plus two minor, phenotypic characteristics of the syndrome (Read & Newton, 1997). The *degree* of presence is unimportant. For example, a small streak of white hair in a dark-haired person is just as clinically significant as an entire head of hair that turned uniformly gray at age 16.

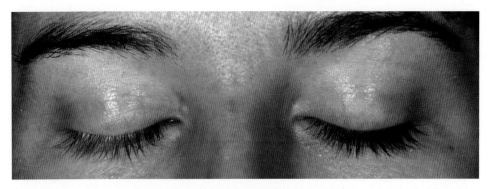

FIGURE 2–1. Subtle differences in pigmentation are just as clinically significant as dramatic pigmentation differences. The eyelashes on the left of the photograph are pale blonde; the eyelashes on the right are dark brown.

Some pigmentation anomalies are very subtle and require careful observation, as in the depigmented eyelashes shown in Figure 2-1.

Although WS1 and WS3 are phenotypically similar, they can result from more than 40 different genetic mutations on chromosome 2 (Nance, 2003). Some researchers consider WS type 3 to be a variation of WS type 1 (Smith, Kolodziej, & Olney, 1998; Wollnik, Tukel, Uyguner, Ghanbari, Kayserili, Emiroglu, & Yukesl-Apak, 2003). Table 2-1 presents the major and minor phenotypic features of WS1 and WS3.

Before describing the features of WS1 and WS3, we need to remember the following about phenotypic observations:

■ It is always possible for someone to have more than one genetic syndrome. In such a case, phenotypic features diagnostic of both syndromes may be present.

■ Not everyone who has WS exhibits all (or even many) of the phenotypic signs of the disorder.

■ A number of medical conditions have phenotypes similar to WS. These conditions, and their differential diagnoses, are discussed in detail in chapter 4.

■ Most of the phenotypic characteristics of WS can be concealed cosmetically. For example, eye color can be changed by contact lenses; hair color can be altered with dyes and wigs. Hearing loss is always invisible, unless the individual is wearing an amplification device. This means we often have to ask patients about original eye and hair color and to be aware of minor features that may cue us to the need to ask these questions.

TABLE 2–1. Phenotypic Features of WS1 and WS3

MAJOR Phenotypic Features of WS

- Heterochromia iridis

- Bright blue eyes

- Dystopia canthorum

- Depigmented head or facial hair

- Congenital sensorineural hearing loss

- Presence of an affected first-degree relative (parent or sibling) with WS

MINOR Phenotypic Features of WS

- Prematurely gray hair

- Congenital leucoderma

- Multiple nevi

- Synophrys

- Hypoplastic nasal alae

- Soft tissue syndactyly of digits

- Polydactyly

- Mandibular hypoplasia

■ People with WS phenotypes often have physical features that are considered desirable (bright blue eyes, for example). Although some individuals with WS are very unusual looking, this is not always the case. The underlying assumption that syndromic individuals must be physically unattractive should be set aside when observing WS phenotypes.

■ Taken individually, many of the features in Table 2-1 are not diagnostic of WS. For example, bright blue eyes, synophrys, and other features are found in numerous syndromes. When we look for the WS phenotype, we are looking for a *pattern of anomalies*. Remember that, by Read and Newton's (1997) standards, an individual must have two major, or one major and two minor, phenotypic characteristics to be considered at risk for WS.

■ People with WS usually have normal cognitive skills. The under-lying assumption held by many health care professionals that syn-dromic individuals must be mentally retarded or developmentally delayed should also be set aside when observing WS phenotypes.

Major Phenotypic Characteristics of WS1

Notice that congenital sensorineural hearing loss and presence of an affected first-degree relative are considered major phenotypic characteristics. This information can be obtained from family interviews, pedigrees, and audiologic testing as described in chapters 4 and 5. The remaining features describe appearance of eyes and hair. These can be noted by careful observation of the patient's head and neck region. Eye anomalies are especially diagnostic of syndromes in general, and WS in particular.

Eye Anomalies

Eye anomalies are common in all types of WS. These usually are anomalies of eye *appearance,* not vision. Most individuals with WS have normal vision, although amblyopia and strabismus are sometimes present. The wide, flat-tened nasal bridge and dystopia canthorum characteristic of WS may cause individuals to appear to have strabismus, when in fact they do not.

The two most clinically significant eye anomalies for diagnosing WS are heterochromia iridis, and bright blue eyes. Heterochromia means "different color," and "iridis" refer to the iris, or colored part of the eye. People with het-erochromia iridis may have two different colored eyes (one brown eye and one blue eye, for example), or they may have one eye that is significantly darker than the other (one light brown eye and one dark brown eye, for example). Heterochromia iridis can also mean that there are two different colors in the same eye, as in the eye examples in Figure 2–2. People with heterochromia iridis may develop the unusual eye coloration shortly after birth or the pigment change may occur later in life. Heterochromia may be so slight that it is only observable in certain lighting conditions, or when the individual is wearing clothing that approximates the color of the darker eye. The woman in Figure 2–3 is a public school teacher. She reports that her students often notice the difference in the color of her eyes, but that her own sister was not aware of the anomaly until she and her sister were teenagers. Heterochromia has many possible causes besides WS. Look for a *pattern of anomalies* when observing phenotypic characteristics. Heterochromia may or may not be a part of the pattern. Keep the whole picture in mind when making clinical phenotypic observations.

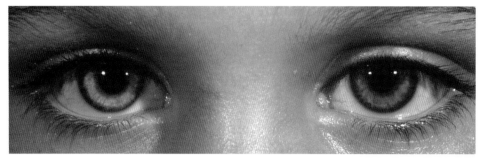

A.

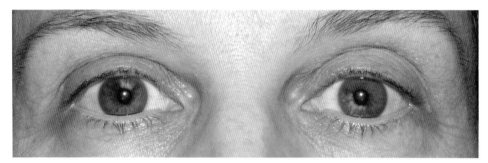

B.

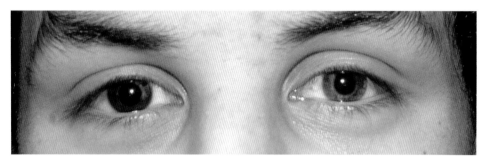

C.

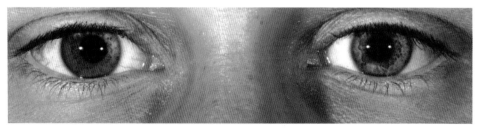

D.

FIGURE 2–2. Heterochromia may take several forms. The eyes in **A.** are two completely different colors. The photographs in **B.** and **C.** show heterochromia in a mother (*B*) and her teenaged son (*C*). Both experienced eye color change from blue to patchy brown around the time of puberty. When heterochromia occurs as an isolated feature, as it does in the eye shown in **D.**, it is impossible to know if it is a phenotypic sign of WS, a sign of another syndrome with heterochromia as a feature, or if it is just an interesting pigmentation anomaly.

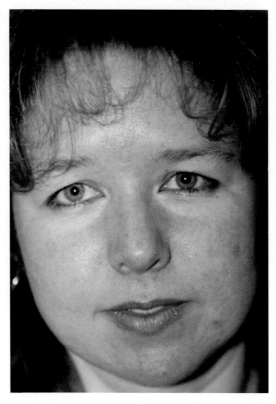

FIGURE 2–3. Heterochromia, like other pigment differences, may be very subtle, and may go unnoticed by the casual observer. This young woman has a blue eye, and a darker blue-gray eye. The difference in color is more noticeable when she wears blue clothing.

Bright blue eyes are also characteristic of someone with WS (Figure 2–4A and 2–4B). This eye color is very beautiful and is often not recognized as a sign of a genetic syndrome, at least by the family members of the person with blue eyes. Blue eyes in combination with prematurely gray hair, or blue eyes and a white streak of hair in the forehead, suggest WS. Blue eyes are characteristic of many syndromes, as well as being a common eye color in certain ethnic groups. We often need to distinguish which blue eyes are diagnostic and which are appropriate to an individual's background. The information in the shaded box on the next page is included to help you understand the relationship of pigment to blue eye problems in general and to serve as a reference for differential diagnosis.

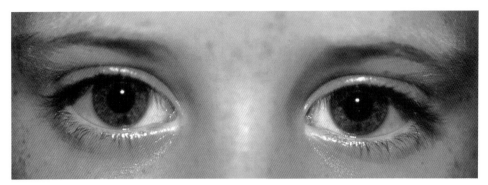

A.

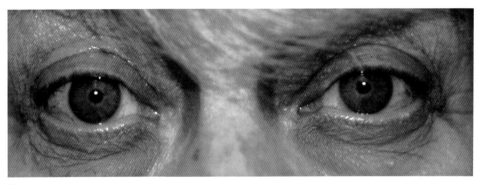

B.

FIGURE 2–4. A. Beautiful, bright blue eyes are characteristic phenotypic features of WS. **B.** Bright blue eyes in an older individual with WS.

Blue-Eye Facts

■ All babies are born with blue eyes regardless of race or ethnic background. After birth an additional pigment layer darkens into the baby's final eye color (unless the baby is going to have blue eyes as an adult).

■ Eye trauma can destroy the overlying darker pigment and expose the underlying blue pigment. Sometimes this condition appears similar to heterochromia iridis.

■ Blue eyes usually result from a recessive inheritance pattern. This means that for an individual to inherit blue eyes he or she must receive a recessive blue eye gene from both parents.

■ Individuals with blue eyes often have ancestors who originated in cold countries that have low exposure to sunshine. The pigment in skin, hair, and eyes is typically lighter in individuals whose ancestors originated in cold climates. Swedes, Norwegians, and Germans are ethnic groups whose members tend to have blue or light-colored eyes. Persons whose ancestors came from hot climates near the high sunshine levels of the equator usually have dark hair, skin, and eyes, because pigment is designed to protect our skin and eyes from sunlight.

■ Individuals with blue eyes are often photophobic and experience discomfort when their eyes are exposed to strong light. Dark-eyed individuals, on the other hand, have extra pigment that protects their eyes from bright light. The woman in Figure 2–5 has light blue eyes that are extremely light sensitive. This photograph was taken on a cloudy day, under the overhanging porch of a building. Despite the dim conditions, and despite the fact that a camera flash was not used, she experienced discomfort during the photography session. Photophobia can also be caused by congenital cataracts. Photophobia is not characteristic of WS, but may be present if the individual with WS has very pale or very light blue eyes or has other eye disorders unrelated to WS. Individuals who experience photophobia should be referred to an ophthalmologist for diagnosis and treatment.

■ Individuals with blue eyes often have poor night vision.

■ Many genetic syndromes and medical conditions have blue eyes as a phenotypic characteristic. The following are syndromes in which blue eyes are a common phenotypic feature: Angelman syndrome (pale blue), ectrodactyly-ectodermal dysplasia-clefting (EEC) syndrome, fragile X syndrome (pale blue), Prader-Willi syndrome, albinism, and Waardenburg syndrome (bright blue with or without heterochromia iridis).

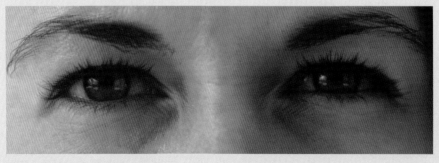

FIGURE 2–5. Photophobia, or visual discomfort when eyes are exposed to bright lights, is often characteristic of blue eyes.

Mid-Face Anomalies

After observing eye color, observe the mid-face for anomalies indicating WS. The *mid-face* extends from the eyebrows to the lower lip and is a common site for WS types 1 and 3 anomalies to occur. These anomalies include decreased nasal bone and philtrum length, and dystopia canthorum. The child in Figure 2–6 has several mid-facial anomalies common in persons with WS Types 1 and 3. Notice that the child's eyes appear unusually widely set and that they give a "cross-eyed" look to the boy's face. The inner corners (canthi) of the eyes are displaced laterally, and the skin from the nasal bridge produces prominent epicanthal folds. The false appearance of strabismus is caused by the folds of skin that obscure the inner corner of both eyes. This condition is called *dystopia canthorum*. Dystopia canthorum is often the most penetrant feature of WS1. Dystopia canthorum can be measured using a formula called the W Index. Read and Newton (1997) give detailed instructions for using this formula, which requires measuring the inner canthal, interpupillary, and outer canthal distances of the eyes. The resulting number, if greater than 2.07 suggests the presence of WS1. Compare the appearance of the child with WS1 in Figure 2–6 with a nonsyndromic Asian individual in Figure 2–7. Notice that

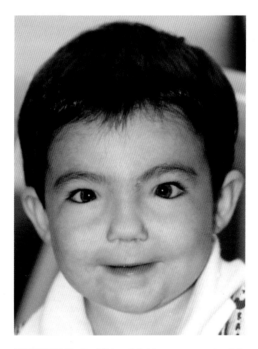

FIGURE 2–6. This child has several mid-facial anomalies common to individuals with WS Type 1. These include hypoplastic nasal alae, small nares, synophrys, bright blue eyes, and dystopia canthorum.

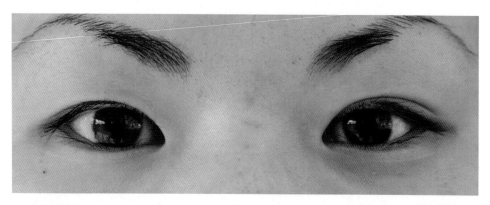

FIGURE 2–7. Appearance of epicanthal folds in a normal Asian individual.

the child in Figure 2-6 has normal eyes, but an unusually broad nasal root. The bones of the nasal bridge in this child are broad and flattened. Because the nasal bridge bones are flat, the skin above the nose has little to support it, and it drapes over the inner corners of the eyes producing epicanthal folds. Such folds are a normal feature for Asian individuals (Figure 2-7), because Asians typically have smaller, flatter nasal bridge bones than Caucasian or black individuals. Dystopia canthorum is *not* a normal facial feature for an individual of any race. Visual observation of eye width can be misleading. It is best to take eye measurements to determine if dystopia canthorum is present and to determine if epicanthal folds are a minor anomaly or an indicator of a more serious condition. The child in Figure 2-6 also has bright blue eyes, flared eyebrows, and a profound bilateral sensorineural hearing loss, all of which are indicative of WS type 1.

Figure 2-8 shows the father of the boy in Figure 2-6. He has the major phenotypic features of WS 1, including: first-degree relative with WS 1, congenital sensorineural hearing loss, depigmented scalp hair, dystopia canthorum, and heterochromia iridis. He also has minor phenotypic features of WS, including facial asymmetry, epicanthal folds, patches of depigmented skin on his body, and bushy, flared eyebrows. He also has no sense of smell (anosia).

Mid-face bones of patients with types 1 and 3 WS may be smaller than normal, or incompletely formed. The zygoma (cheekbone) is often smaller than normal, giving the patient's face a flattened appearance in profile (Figure 2-8B).

Hair Anomalies

Pigment is normally extensively present in the hair of normal individuals. Lack of pigment, or early loss of pigment in head hair, is characteristic of several syndromes including Waardenburg. Some individuals with WS have a single white streak of hair above their forehead; others have patches of depigmented hair elsewhere on their head, including eyelashes and sideburns. These depigmented areas may be present at birth or may develop later in life.

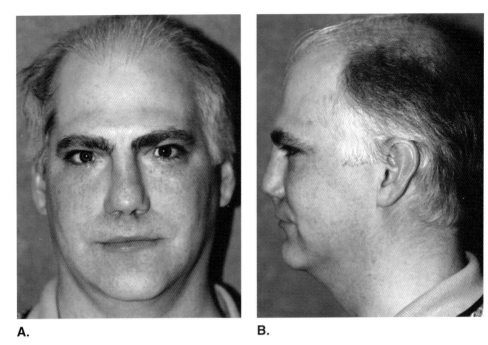

A.   **B.**

FIGURE 2–8. A. An adult male with characteristic features of WS type 1. These include facial asymmetry, heterochromia iridis, epicanthal folds, and a prominent nasal root. This individual has a history of severe headaches. He also has no sense of smell. **B.** Profile of a patient with WS type 1. Notice the flat appearance of the mid-face.

Congenital Sensorineural Hearing Loss

Congenital sensorineural hearing loss is a major, and invisible, characteristic of WS. Like the other phenotypic features of WS, hearing losses associated with the problem may vary in occurrence, location, and degree (Gorlin, Toriello, & Cohen, 1995). Estimates of occurrence of sensorineural hearing losses in WS Type 1 have been variously reported as 20% (Keats, 2002), 36 to 58% (Nayak & Isaacson, 2003), and 20 to 25% (Arnos & Pandya, 2004). The hearing loss may be unilateral or bilateral and may progress as the individual ages. Children with profound congenital sensorineural hearing loss may be good candidates for cochlear implants, as is the child in Figure 2-9.

Minor Phenotypic Characteristics of WS1

Major features of WS are often visually striking and readily observable. Minor features may require more careful observation. These features may occur in the head and neck area, but also on the skin in general, and in the fingers and toes.

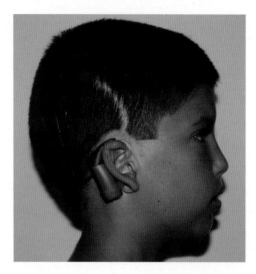

FIGURE 2–9. This child has a profound bilateral hearing loss and has received a cochlear implant. The surgical scar is apparent above his ear. His ear is located in a low position and is slanted toward the back of his head. Such ear positioning is common in individuals with small mandibles, (Photography by Jamie Pratzel.)

Minor Pigmentation Anomalies

Hair is considered prematurely gray if it loses melanin (pigment) before the age of 30. Prematurely gray hair occurs in all types of WS and is often concealed by hair dye. Facial hair as well as head hair may be affected by depigmentation.

Skin also contains melanin. In normal individuals melanin darkens on exposure to sunlight. People with WS often have absence of skin pigment from birth (congenital leucoderma). Depigmented areas of skin do not suntan, are easily sunburned, and are at increased risk for developing skin cancer. Figure 2-10 shows the hand of an individual with WS who has congenital leucoderma of the fingers. These lighter patches of skin have been present from birth and do not darken on exposure to sunlight. Although clinically leucoderma is considered a "minor" feature of WS, persons of color may consider it a major feature. Depigmented areas of skin are more visually striking when they occur on dark-skinned individuals. Because skin color is part of our identity, individuals with pigment anomalies may suffer psychologically and socially when pigment is missing from skin or when pigment is present, but is the "wrong" color for the race of the individual. Individuals with WS who have unusual pigmentation may benefit from psychological counseling

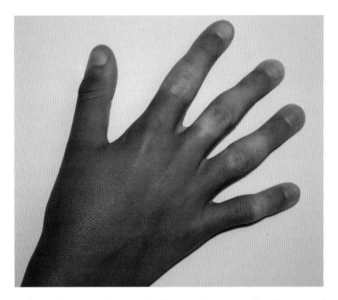

FIGURE 2–10. Congenital leucoderma on the fingers of a boy with WS type 3. (Photography by Jamie Pratzel.)

as well as from cosmetic techniques designed to approximate normal eye, skin, and hair color.

Areas of concentrated pigment also occur on the skin of individuals with WS. Nevi are localized areas of malformed skin usually caused by a concentration of pigment or increased vascularization. Nevi are commonly called "moles," "birthmarks," or "freckles." Nevi may be sprinkled over the entire body, as in the woman in Figure 2-11, and may appear in unusual locations, such as the palms of the hands (Figure 2-12). If the nevus is a vascular tumor of the skin caused by overdevelopment of blood vessels it may appear as a red dot or a large reddish discolored area of skin. When nevi contain melanin, this melanin may grow or darken on exposure to sunlight. Some nevi may become malignant melanomas. People with WS often have large numbers of pigmented nevi on their skin, especially the skin of the head and neck. These nevi should be monitored for changes in size or coloration, and surgically removed if necessary.

Freckles are areas of pigmentation that are randomly distributed on the skin of people with WS (as well as on the skin of people who do not have syndromes). Freckles may cause social embarrassment, but are usually not cause for medical concern.

Synophrys

Synophrys, eyebrows that extend across the bridge of the nose to meet in the midline at the top of the nasal bridge, are considered a minor feature of WS. Notice the presence of synophrys in the boy in Figure 2-13. His eyebrows are also bushy and flared, a common phenotypic finding in all types of WS.

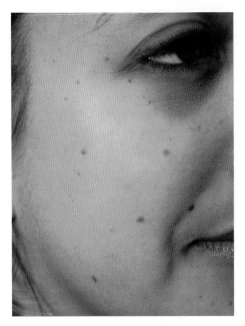

FIGURE 2–11. Multiple nevi on an individual's face. Such nevi are common in patients who have WS, as well as other syndromes.

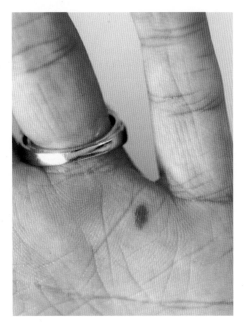

FIGURE 2–12. A nevus located in the palm of the hand. (Photography by Jamie Pratzel.)

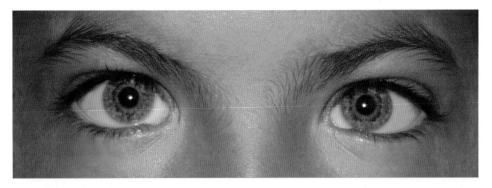

FIGURE 2–13. Bright blue eyes and synophrys are frequent phenotypic features of WS. Some individuals wax the bridge of their nose to remove unwanted facial hair. (Photography by Jamie Pratzel.)

Hypoplastic Nasal Alae

Individuals with WS often have underdeveloped (hypoplastic) facial features. The sides of the tip of the nose (nasal alae) are a common hypoplastic location. All types of WS can produce poorly formed or underdeveloped nasal alae. Figure 2-14 compares a normally developed nose (A) with the nose of a person with WS (B).

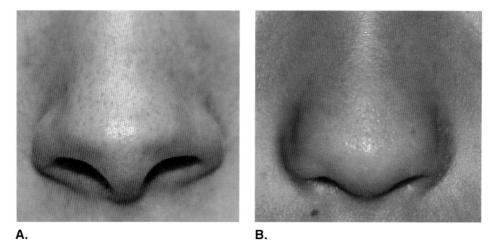

A.   **B.**

FIGURE 2–14. A. Normal noses have well-developed "wings" or lateral edges. **B.** Individuals with WS often have poorly developed nasal alae and small nostrils.

Soft Tissue Syndactyly

Individuals with WS sometimes have minor anomalies of the fingers and toes. Syndactyly is the term for fused fingers or toes. Soft-tissue syndactyly means that the digits are connected by soft tissue (muscles, connective tissue) only, and not by cartilage or bone. Look for signs of syndactyly in fingers or toes, as in the individual in Figure 2–15 who has soft tissue syndactyly of the second and third toes.

Polydactyly

Individuals with WS are occasionally born with extra fingers or toes. These structures are often rudimentary, and can be removed by tying off the digit and stopping the blood supply to the tissue of the extra finger or toe. In time the digit dries up and drops off. Surgery may be needed if the extra fingers and toes contain bone or cartilage. Interestingly, polydactyly can cause more parental concern than the prospect of hearing loss. In terms of health issues polydactyly is usually of minor concern; in terms of emotional connotations, polydactyly can produce a high level of parental anxiety.

Mandibular Hypoplasia

Mandibular hypoplasia is sometimes present in individuals with WS types 1 and 3. Individuals in three of the families under study at our university have family members who exhibit facial asymmetry and small lower jaws. One young woman has undergone plastic reconstructive surgery to reconstruct her mandibles. Although radiography is the most definitive way to identify hypoplastic mandible, it is often possible to recognize the condition by examining or photographing the patient's face in full-face and profile views. Facial asymmetry may be present in full-face view if mandibular hypoplasia is unilateral. Such patients may also complain of temporomandibular joint (TMJ) pain and present with a history of headaches. Individuals with hypoplastic mandibles may also have a receding chin (retrognathic mandible), and their outer ears may slant backward and be placed low on the side of their heads. Figure 2–16 shows a woman with WS and a retrognathic mandible (receding chin), and deafness.

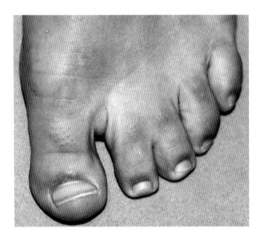

FIGURE 2–15. Soft tissue syndactyly of the second and third toes. Syndactyly of digits is a common occurrence in many syndromes. Look for a pattern of anomalies before assuming that syndactyly indicates the presence of WS.

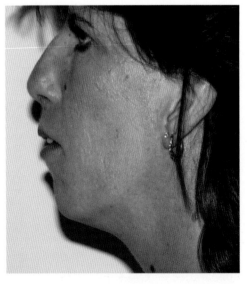

FIGURE 2–16. Retrognathic profile (receding chin) in a woman with WS.

Occasional Anomalies

Individuals with WS 1 and 3 occasionally have other serious medical conditions, including cleft lip and/or cleft palate, spina bifida, anophthalmia, and communication problems secondary to cleft palate and hearing loss.

Cleft Lip and/or Cleft Palate

Cleft lip and cleft palate are two separate conditions resulting from developmental errors during the fifth to eighth week in utero. This is the time during which the structures of the face and oral cavity begin to fuse and form. Although the causes of cleft lip and cleft palate are not well understood, these conditions sometimes occur in conjunction with genetic syndromes, including WS. Individuals with cleft lip and/or cleft palate are at risk for a variety of communication disorders, including hearing loss, language delay, and voice, articulation, and resonance problems. Infants with WS and cleft palate benefit from craniofacial team treatment. Figure 2–17 shows a young woman who has undergone team treatment for a unilateral cleft lip and cleft palate as a child. Surgical outcomes vary depending on the nature and extent of the facial anomaly. In this case, the outcome was a near-normal, attractive facial appearance.

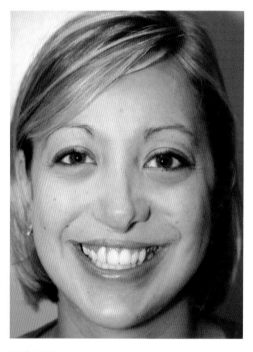

FIGURE 2–17. Post team-treatment appearance of a young woman who was born with unilateral cleft lip and cleft palate.

Spina Bifida

The human spinal cord forms between the 18th to the 30th day in utero. Genetic problems (including WS), lack of folic acid, and other causes can interfere with spinal cord formation and produce birth anomalies including spina bifida (open spine) and anencephaly (absence of the brain and spinal cord). As you take a case history from someone suspected of having WS, remember to ask about stillbirths and infants who failed to survive childhood. Ask about the occurrence of spina bifida, anencephaly, and hydrocephalus in family members. People with WS seldom know the relationship between spinal problems and WS and, therefore, may fail to mention them when relating the family history.

Communication Problems

WS may be accompanied by communication problems, especially if the individual has cleft palate and/or sensorineural hearing loss. The diagnosis and treatment of individuals with sensorineural hearing loss will be discussed in chapter 5.

Although individuals with cleft palate are predisposed by their anatomic condition to develop disorders of speech, language, and resonance, development of communication problems is by no means certain. Early detection and treatment by a competent surgeon and craniofacial team and early intervention by a speech-language pathologist are often sufficient to prevent the development of speech and language problems. If hearing loss accompanies cleft palate, the prognosis for avoiding communication problems becomes more guarded.

Having learned the major and minor phenotypic features of WS type 1, we now can observe them in members of two families of individuals with WS type 1.

PHENOTYPIC FEATURES IN A FAMILY WITH PROBABLE WS TYPE 1

The following individuals have a family history of hearing loss, and the phenotypic features of WS type 1, although the family has not yet had genetic testing to make the diagnosis certain. Figures 2–18A through 2–18E show a woman and her four children. Notice that she (A) shows evidence of prematurely gray hair, hypoplastic nasal alae, small nares, and broad nasal root. She has brown eyes and normal hearing.

Figure 2–18B shows the older daughter. As an infant she had a hemangioma on her left eyelid, which subsequently disappeared. She has brown eyes, normal hearing, bushy eyebrows, downslanting palpebral fissures (indicating midface hypoplasia), and multiple nevi.

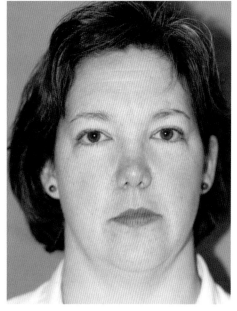

A.

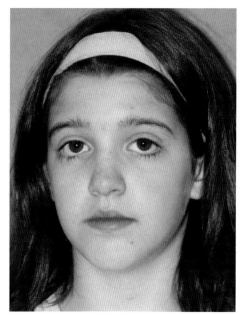

B.

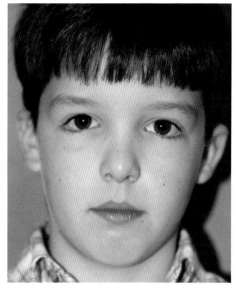

C.

FIGURE 2–18. A family with phenotypic features of WS type 1. The mother **A.** has prematurely gray hair in her forehead, hypoplastic nasal alae, small nares, and a broad nasal root. Her hearing is normal. The oldest child **B.** also has normal hearing, hypoplastic nasal alae, and broad nasal root. The second child **C.** has flared eyebrows, hypoplastic nasal alae, small nares, multiple nevi, and a broad nasal root. His hearing is normal. *(continues)*

The boy in Figure 2–18C also has mid-face hypoplasia, downslanting palpebral fissures, flared eyebrows, hypoplastic nasal alae, multiple nevi, and normal hearing. He also has only one kidney. The congenital kidney anomaly is unrelated to WS, as kidney anomalies are not part of the phenotype for individuals with WS.

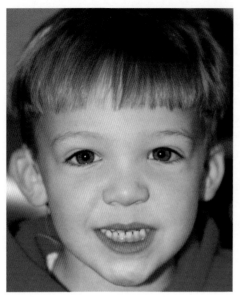 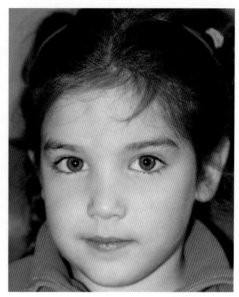

D.   **E.**

FIGURE 2–18. *(continued)* The third child **D.** has blue eyes, a broad nasal root, hypoplastic mid-face, and is profoundly deaf. The youngest child **E.** has flared eyebrows, broad nasal root, hypoplastic nasal alae, and normal hearing.

Figure 2–18D shows the youngest boy, a profoundly deaf child with blue-gray eyes. He has received a cochlear implant and has achieved near-normal age-appropriate speech development. As a baby he had very pronounced epicanthal folds. The family did not discover the likelihood that they had WS1 until the birth of this child. The child's hearing loss was not discovered until he failed to develop normal speech. He also has a renal anomaly unrelated to WS.

The girl in Figure 2–18E is the family's youngest child. She has blue eyes, flared eyebrows, hypoplastic nasal alae, and normal hearing.

PHENOTYPIC CHARACTERISTICS OF WS TYPE 3

WS Type 3 is named *Klein-Waardenburg syndrome* after David Klein, a physician who assisted Petrus Waardenburg to fully understand WS by introducing him to a patient who had severe musculoskeletal anomalies as well as evidence of pigmentary features common to WS (Read & Newton, 1997). Individuals with WS 3 may be expected to have any or all of the major or minor phenotypic characteristics of individuals with WS 1. In addition, they have anomalies of the upper limbs and, very rarely, anophthalmia. Hypoplastic upper limbs, profound hearing loss, and severe depigmentation occur frequently in WS Type 3. Minor contractures of the elbows or fingers may also occur sporadically.

Anophthalmia

Anophthalmia is a very rare condition that is sometimes found in individuals with WS type 3. Le Merrer et al. (1988) referred to individuals who had WS in conjunction with anomalies of the hands, feet, and eyes as ophthalmo-acromelic syndrome. Eye anomalies range from mild microphthalmia (small eye) to complete anophthalmia (absence of the eyes). This condition is extremely rare, and is autosomal recessive. Parental consanguinity is believed to be responsible for the increased incidence of ophthalmo-acromelic syndrome in Turkey (Suyugul et al., 1996). These individuals are usually identified early in life and are best referred to a craniofacial team for long-term treatment.

Although the phenotypic features of WS1 and WS3 are similar, there are minor differences. The shaded box below compares basic information about WS Types 1 and 3.

Comparison of WS Types 1 and 3

Inheritance Pattern and Gene Locus WS Types 1 and 3
Autosomal dominant, 2q35

Inheritance Pattern of Ophthalmo-Acromelic Syndrome (Subtype of WS 3)
Autosomal recessive

Prenatal Diagnosis
Available for both WS1 and WS3

Hearing Loss
WS Type 1: congenital, variable sensorineural hearing loss
WS Type 3: progressive sensorineural hearing loss

Major Anomalies of WS Types 1 and 3
- Heterochromia iridis
- Bright blue eyes
- Dystopia canthorum
- Depigmented hair
- Congenital sensorineural hearing loss

Minor Anomalies of WS Types 1 and 3
- Prematurely gray hair
- Congenital leucoderma
- Multiple nevi

- Synophrys
- Hypoplastic nasal alae
- Mandibular hypoplasia

Occasional Anomalies WS Types 1 and 3
- Speech and language problems secondary to cleft palate and sensorineural hearing loss
- Cleft palate
- Spina bifida

Major Anomalies WS Type 3
- Upper limb anomalies

Minor Anomalies WS Type 3
- Minor joint contractures

Occasional Anomalies of WS Type 3
- Anophthalmia and limb defects (ophthalmo-acromelic syndrome)

PHENOTYPIC FEATURES IN A FAMILY WITH PROBABLE WS TYPE 3

Figure 2-19 shows a mother and son who have WS type 3. This woman's parents were deaf. Her father has WS3 and a profound, bilateral, sensorineural hearing loss. He communicated using both sign language and oral language. His hair went prematurely gray at the age of 25.

His daughter and grandson (Figure 2-19) also have WS3. His daughter was unaware that she and her father had WS until her son was born and genetic testing was done. She has heterochromia; unilateral, severe sensorineural hearing loss; a history of amblyopia; and musculoskeletal anomalies. Her hair became prematurely gray at age 16. Her hands have pronounced camptodactyly (Figure 2-20). Her siblings have received genetic testing and do not have the gene for WS3.

Her son (Figure 2-21) was born with a moderate to severe, bilateral sensorineural hearing loss. Despite amplification and speech therapy, he was unable to communicate orally. At age one he received surgery to correct strabismus and is expected to have additional surgery to correct the problem. He has had frequent bouts of otitis media, and wears pressure equalization (PE) tubes. He has camptodactyly, leucoderma of the hand, narrow shoulders with underdeveloped muscles, and multiple nevi. He received a cochlear implant

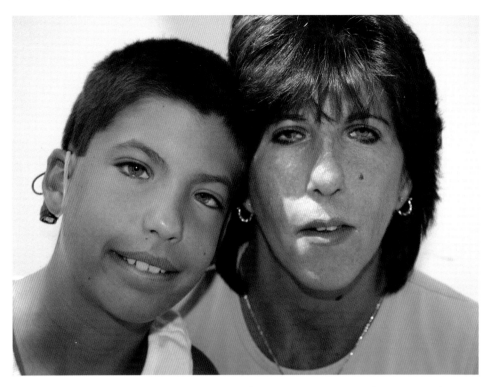

FIGURE 2–19. A mother and son with WS type 3. The mother has heterochromia iridis, hypoplastic nasal alae, neck webbing, and a severe, unilateral, sensorineural hearing loss in her fight ear. She covers her prematurely gray hair with hair dye. Notice the mole on her cheek. (Photography by Jamie Pratzel.)

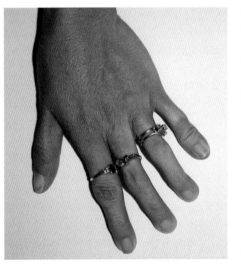

A.

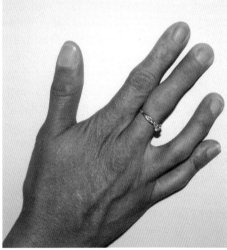

B.

FIGURE 2–20. Camptodactyly, or contracted digits, is a phenotypic characteristic of WS type 3. This feature is visible in the little fingers of both hands in this adult with WS3. (Photography by Jamie Pratzel.)

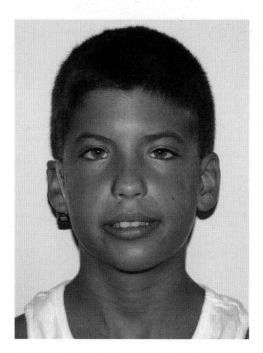

FIGURE 2–21. This boy with WS3 shows characteristic underdevelopment of shoulder muscles. He also exhibits blue eyes, synophrys, hypoplastic nasal alae, and is profoundly deaf. (Photography by Jamie Pratzel.)

in his right ear when he was 3½ years old. He was diagnosed with attention deficit disorder at 5½ years of age. During that time he began to attend an oral/auditory institute for the deaf. He began to develop oral speech at age 6 and continues to use oral speech for communication.

A FAMILY WITH FEATURES OF WS OF UNKNOWN TYPE

The family described below is a good example of a family that is aware that hearing loss "runs in the family," but until recently was unaware that the hearing loss is probably syndrome related. Features of WS have appeared in four generations of the family in the form of hearing loss, asymmetric facies, blue eyes, and, recently, polydactyly. The family also has incidences of neural tube defects and cleft palate and cleft lip. Figure 2-22A shows a woman with unilateral profound hearing loss, blue eyes, hypoplastic mandibles, facial asymmetry, and mild balance problems. She has learned to compensate for her hearing loss, and except for difficulty in locating the direction of sounds,

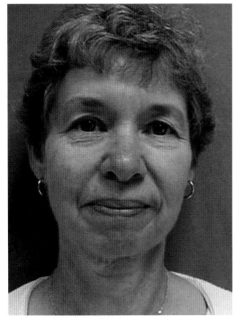

A.

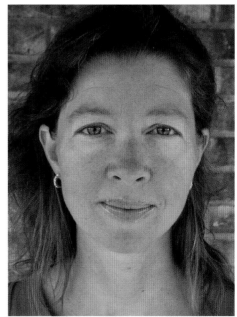

B.

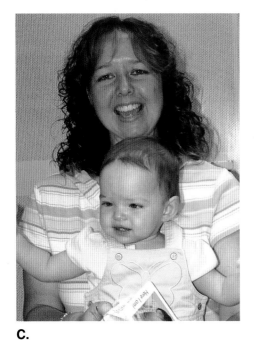

C.

FIGURE 2–22. A family with phenotypic features of WS of unknown type. **A.** A woman with a unilateral profound hearing loss, blue eyes, hypoplastic mandibles, facial asymmetry and mild balance problems. **B.** Her oldest daughter who has facial asymmetry, TMJ pain, frequent headaches, and normal hearing. **C.** The mother's younger daughter, and her granddaughter. Both the daughter and granddaughter have normal hearing, although both show phenotypic features of WS.

experiences few hearing-related problems. The woman in Figure 2–22B is her older daughter who has facial asymmetry, TMJ pain, frequent debilitating headaches, and hypothyroidism. Her hearing is normal. Figure 2–22C is the younger daughter. She has slight facial asymmetry, heterochromia that is more noticeable under certain conditions, and normal hearing. Her daughter (Figure 2–22C) has red hair, bright blue eyes, amblyopia, and was born with bilateral postaxial polydactyly. Because of the family history of (probable) WS-related hearing loss, the infant was tested at the Miami University Speech and Hearing Clinic with a battery of hearing tests including otoacoustic emissions (OAEs). Her hearing is normal.

SUMMARY

In this chapter you have learned:

■ The major and minor phenotypic characteristics of WS types 1 and 3.

■ The major features that distinguish WS Type 1 from WS type 3.

The following chapter will discuss the genotypic and phenotypic characteristics of WS types 2 and 4.

REFERENCES

Arnos, K. S., & Pandya, A. (2004). Genes for deafness and the genetics program at Gallaudet University. In J. V. Van Cleve (Ed.), *Genetics, disability, and deafness* (pp. 111–126). Washington, DC: Gallaudet University Press.

Gorlin, R. J., Toriello, H. V., & Cohen, M. M. (1995). *Hereditary hearing loss and its syndromes.* Oxford: Oxford University Press.

Keats, B. J. (2002). Genes and syndromic hearing loss. *Journal of Communication Disorders, 35,* 355–366.

Le Merrer, M., Nessmann, C., Briad, M. L., & Maroteaux, P. (1988). Ophthalmoacromelic syndrome. *Annals of Genetics, 31,* 226–229.

Nance, W. E. (2003). The genetics of deafness. *Mental Retardation and Developmental Disabilities Research Reviews, 9,* 109–119.

Nayak, C. S., & Isaacson, G. (2003). Worldwide distribution of Waardenburg syndrome. *Annals of Otology, Rhinolology, and Laryngology, 112,* 817–820.

Read, A., & Newton, V. (1997). Waardenburg syndrome. *Journal of Medical Genetics, 34,* 656–665.

Smith, S., Kolodziej, P., & Olney, A. H. (1998). Waardenburg syndrome. *Ear, Nose, and Throat Journal, 77*(4), 257–258.

Suyugul, Z., Seven, M., Hacihanefioglu, S., Kartal, A., Suyugul, N., & Cenani, A. (1996). Anophthalmia-Waardenburg syndrome: A report of three cases. *American Journal of Medical Genetics, 62,* 391–397.

Toriello, H. V., Reardon, W., & Gorlin, R. J. (Eds.). (2004). *Hereditary hearing loss and its syndromes.* Oxford: Oxford University Press.

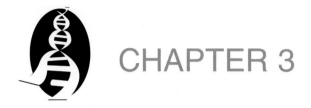

CHAPTER 3

Waardenburg Syndrome Types 2 and 4

Waardenburg syndrome types 2 and 4 have phenotypes similar to types 1 and 3, but with some major differences:

■ Neither WS2 nor WS4 presents with dystopia canthorum or musculoskeletal anomalies.

■ WS2 may have ocular albinism as a phenotypic feature.

■ WS type 4 has the additional disorder of Hirschsprung's disease (HD) associated with it.

After reading this chapter you should be able to:

■ Compare the phenotypic characteristics of WS types 1 and 3 with the phenotypic characteristics of WS types 2 and 4.

■ Describe the health implications for someone who has ocular albinism.

■ Describe the type of hearing loss that accompanies WS types 2 and 4.

■ Name the type of inheritance patterns for WS types 2 and 4.

■ Describe the health implications for someone who has Hirschsprung's disease.

WS TYPE 2

WS type 2 has several subtypes, each of which have specific gene loci, and specific types of inheritance patterns (see shaded box). The majority of anomalies common to WS types 1 and 3 are present in WS type 2, with the *exception* of dystopia canthorum and musculoskeletal anomalies. Table 3-1 compares the major and minor phenotypic features of WS2 and WS4.

TABLE 3–1. Phenotypic Features of WS2 and WS4

MAJOR Phenotypic Features of WS2

- Heterochromia iridis
- Congenital sensorineural hearing loss
- Presence of an affected first-degree relative (parent or sibling) with WS
- Bright blue eyes
- Depigmented head or facial hair

MAJOR Phenotypic Features of WS4

- Hirschsprung's disease (HD)
- Heterochromia iridis
- Congenital sensorineural hearing loss
- Presence of an affected first-degree relative (parent or sibling) with WS
- Bright blue eyes
- Depigmented head or facial hair

MINOR Phenotypic Features of WS2 and WS4

- Prematurely gray hair
- Congenital leucoderma
- Multiple nevi
- Synophrys
- Hypoplastic nasal alae
- Soft tissue syndactyly of digits
- Polydactyly
- Mandibular hypoplasia

Comparison of WS Types 2 and 4

Inheritance Pattern and Gene Locus of WS2A

Generalized Hypopigmentation (Tietz syndrome)
Autosomal dominant
3p14.1–p12.3

Prenatal Diagnosis
Available

Major Anomalies for *all* types of WS2
- Heterochromia iridis
- Bright blue eyes
- Depigmented hair
- Congenital sensorineural hearing loss

Minor Anomalies for *all* types of WS2
- Prematurely gray hair
- Congenital leucoderma
- Multiple nevi
- Synophrys
- Hypoplastic nasal alae
- Mandibular hypoplasia

Inheritance Pattern and Gene Locus of WS2B
Autosomal dominant
1p21–p13.3

Prenatal Diagnosis
Not available

Major and Minor Anomalies
See above

Inheritance Pattern and Gene Locus of WS2C
Autosomal dominant
8p23

Prenatal Diagnosis
Not available

Major Anomalies and Minor Anomalies
See above

Inheritance Pattern and Gene Locus of WS2D
Autosomal recessive
Deletions of SLUG transcription factor 8q11

Prenatal Diagnosis
Not available

Major Anomalies
See above

Inheritance Pattern and Gene Locus of WS2 with Ocular Albinism
Autosomal digenic
Xp11.4–p11.23

Prenatal Diagnosis
Not available

Major and Minor Anomalies
Above anomalies plus ocular albinism

Inheritance Pattern and Gene Locus of WS type 4 (Shah-Waardenburg syndrome)
Autosomal recessive
20q13.2–q13.3
Autosomal dominant
SOX locus on chromosome 22q13 and 13q22

Major and Minor Anomalies
Same as above *with* Hirschsprung's disease (HD)

HETEROCHROMIA IRIDIS

Heterochromia iridis occurs frequently in WS2 and WS4, with occurrence rates of 47% of patients with WS2 (Dourmishev et al., 1999). The appearance of heterochromia iridis is similar to that occurring in WS1 and WS3.

SENSORINEURAL HEARING LOSS

The incidence of sensorineural hearing loss in WS2 has been variously reported as 77% (Dourmishev et al., 1999) and 87% (Griffith & Friedman, 2002). The variability in reported incidence of hearing loss is compounded because some studies include mild and moderate sensorineural hearing losses in their reports, whereas others report only the incidence of severe to profound sensorineural losses. Arnos and Pandya (2004) state that deafness occurs in 50% of individuals with WS type 2.

WS2 WITH OCULAR ALBINISM

Some individuals who have WS2 also have reduced pigment in their eyes as well as abnormal development of the retina and/or nerve connections between the eyes and the brain. This condition is called ocular albinism. Sometimes the individual also has depigmented skin and hair (oculocutaneous albinism). Both conditions can be diagnosed by an eye exam. Oculocutaneous albinism occurs in several syndromes and is not specifically diagnostic of WS2. Remember that phenotypic diagnosis of WS requires a *pattern of characteristics* suggestive of the syndrome. Individuals who have ocular albinism often have pale blue irises and reduced retinal pigment. Lack of pigment causes reduced visual acuity and heightened sensitivity to bright light. Strabismus (crossed eyes) and nystagmus are also features of ocular albinism, and are discussed more fully in chapter 4. Individuals who have WS and ocular albinism may have low vision, and may be sensitive to bright lights and glare. Any patient exhibiting these features should be referred for examination and treatment by an ophthalmologist, preferably one with knowledge of and interest in genetically caused vision problems. These patients may also need special assistance to read and to perform daily activities requiring good vision.

Not all individuals with WS2 have ocular albinism. WS2 must be differentially diagnosed by a combination of genetic testing, pedigree development, vision testing, and phenotypic examination. WS2 is a severe form of Waardenburg syndrome because of its associated dual sensory problems.

PHENOTYPIC FEATURES IN A FAMILY WITH
WAARDENBURG TYPE 2

Three generations of this family have presented with phenotypic signs of WS2. Figure 3–1 shows a woman with bright blue eyes, prematurely gray hair, and normal hearing. She has multiple nevi, and lacks the broad, flat, nasal

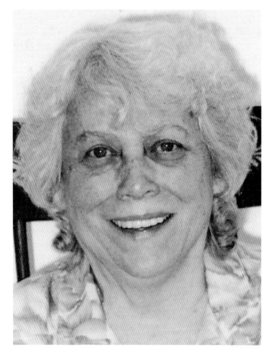

FIGURE 3–1. A woman with WS2, prematurely gray hair, and bright blue eyes.

bridge and dystopia canthorum found in WS types 1 and 3. Her daughter (Figure 3-2) has heterochromia, flaring eyebrows, and prematurely gray hair, which she conceals with hair dye. She has normal hearing. Her son (Figure 3-3) was born with a profound unilateral hearing loss. This was the first time the family became aware of the relationship between their physical appearance and hearing loss. This young man has heterochromia, multiple nevi, and flared eyebrows. Other members of the extended family also have phenotypic signs of WS2.

WS TYPE 4 (SHAH-WAARDENBURG SYNDROME)

Individuals with WS4 may exhibit any or all of the major or minor characteristics of individuals with WS2 in addition to Hirschsprung's disease, also called Hirschsprung's megacolon or aganglionic megacolon. Because this condition is usually manifested shortly after birth, and may be life-threatening, WS4 is considered a potentially lethal syndrome. WS4 occurs in families, and also spontaneously. Familial forms are sometimes associated with consanguinity.

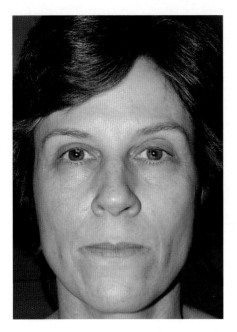

FIGURE 3–2. Heterochromia iridis and flaring eyebrows in a woman with WS2.

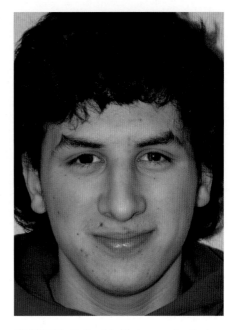

FIGURE 3–3. Multiple nevi, flaring eyebrows, and heterochromia in a young man with WS2.

Hirschsprung's Disease (HD)

Hirschsprung's disease is a congenital disease of the large intestine (colon) that causes chronic constipation. During fetal development nerve cells called ganglion cells develop in the small intestine and continue developing along the length of the large intestine. Ganglion cells cause the muscle contractions in the bowels that move feces through the intestines and out of the body. If ganglion cells are missing from the large intestine, the disease is called aganglionic megacolon, or HD. Sometimes the small intestine also lacks ganglion cells. This condition is called long-segment disease.

Children who are born with HD develop an enlarged colon, chronic constipation, and failure to thrive. If HD is not diagnosed and treated immediately, intestinal infection, rupture of the colon, or death may occur. HD is managed by "pull-through" surgical procedures in which the aganglionic section of intestines is removed, and the healthy section attached to the rectum. The longer the aganglionic segment, the higher the risk for an unsuccessful outcome. As with ocular albinism, HD alone is not diagnostic of WS4. HD occurs in several other syndromes (see sidebar), each with specific genetic loci.

Although HD is a serious, sometimes lethal, condition, individuals are usually able to lead normal lives following corrective surgery. Depending on treatment outcome, individuals may need special diets, tube feeding,

---

Syndromes with HD as a Feature

- Down syndrome (Trisomy 21)
- Smith-Lemli-Opitz syndrome
- Ondine-Hirschsprung disease
- Cartilage-hair hypoplasia.
- WS type 4

HD mutations have been mapped to a number of locations including:

- Xq28
- 20q13.2–q13.3
- 19p13.3
- 10q11.2
- 5p13.1–p12
- 4p12

HD is potentially life-threatening.

---

additional fluid intake, and monitoring for constipation, diarrhea, and/or infection. Support organizations for individuals with HD are included in chapter 4.

SUMMARY

As clinicians, we need to understand the major differences between types of WS because these differences impact development of treatment plans and prognoses for treatment outcomes. WS2 and WS4 are very serious, sometimes lethal, forms of Waardenburg's syndrome. WS2 and WS4 have phenotypes similar to individuals with WS types 1 and 3. However, WS2 and WS4 do not have dystopia canthorum or musculoskeletal anomalies associated with them. The *additional features* of ocular albinism (WS2) and Hirschsprung's disease (WS4) can produce severe health problems, dual sensory disorders, heightened risk of skin cancer, and other complications. Ocular albinism and HD are also features of several syndromes, so differential diagnosis of patients with these medical conditions is vital for treatment success and for predicting the occurrence of the conditions in future generations. In this chapter you have learned:

■ The major and minor phenotypic characteristics of WS types 2 and 4.

■ The major features that distinguish WS type 2 from WS type 4.

■ The diagnostic manifestations of ocular albinism.

■ The characteristics of Hirschsprung's disease, and its relationship to WS type 4.

In the following chapter you will learn how WS and its related anomalies are diagnosed, and how WS is distinguished from similar genetic syndromes and skin conditions.

REFERENCES

Arnos, K. S., & Pandya, A. (2004). Genes for deafness and the genetics program at Gallaudet University. In J. V. Van Cleve (Ed.), *Genetics, disability, and deafness* (pp. 111–126). Washington, DC: Gallaudet University Press.

Dourmishev, A., Dourmishev, L., Schwartz, R., & Janniger, C. (1999). Waardenburg syndrome. *International Journal of Dermatology, 38,* 656–663.

Griffith, A. J., & Friedman, T. B. (2002). Autosomal and X-linked auditory disorders. In B. J. B. Keats, A. N. Popper, & R. R. Fay (Eds.). *Genetics and auditory disorders* (pp. 121–127). Berlin, Germany: Springer-Verlag.

Nayak, C. S., & Isaacson, G. (2003). Worldwide distribution of Waardenburg syndrome. *Annals of Otology, Rhinology, and Laryngology, 112,* 817–820.

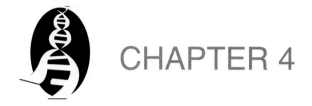

CHAPTER 4

Differential Diagnosis of Waardenburg Syndrome

*C*hapter 1 described several ways that scientists diagnose genetic syndromes. This chapter addresses the specific application of these diagnostic methods to Waardenburg syndrome, and compares the characteristics of WS to those of similar conditions and syndromes. It also reviews diagnostic techniques for assessing the problems associated with WS. After reading this chapter you should be able to:

■ Explain why individuals and families of individuals with WS may be unaware of a genetic basis for their WS-related physical problems.

■ List the advantages and limitations of using phenotype to diagnose WS.

■ List three genetic conditions that may easily be mistaken for WS.

■ Explain the relevance of family history and pedigree to diagnosing WS.

■ Define the role of an audiologist in diagnosing WS.

■ Describe the advantages and limitations of genotyping in diagnosing WS.

■ Define the role of a genetic counselor in diagnosing WS.

■ Define the role of a craniofacial team in the diagnostic process.

■ Define the role of a speech-language pathologist in diagnosing WS.

RECOGNIZING GENETIC PROBLEMS

A problem must be recognized before it can be diagnosed. Visual and auditory evidence of genetic problems is all around us. We can see it in our patients' faces, hear it in coworkers' speech and voices, observe it in the behavior of strangers on the street, and sometimes see it reflected in a mirror. The first step in diagnosing WS is to train ourselves to observe syndromic implications, even if the evidence is subtle, or, in the case of hearing loss, invisible. It might seem that anyone would immediately notice the phenotypic signs of WS, because for the most part they are visually striking. Hearing loss, when present, is often severe and affects the patient's communicative ability in a variety of ways. However, my experience in working with families of patients with WS contradicts the assumption that individuals with WS know they have a genetic syndrome. The following statement by the mother of a child with WS type 3 summarizes the effect of a definitive diagnosis on the patient's perception of her facial anomalies and hearing loss.

> When my son was one year old, an audiologist suspected that my son and I had WS due to our facial features and hearing loss. We underwent genetic counseling to verify that we did have WS Type 3. Based on pictures of my father, it was suspected that he also had WS. Receiving this diagnosis somehow helped me to deal with our differences. Until then, I never knew what caused my facial anomalies and hearing loss. Knowing the cause of our differences has helped me to accept them.

In this family's case, knowledge of a genetic syndrome ultimately led to understanding, treatment, and acceptance of the effects of WS. The suggestion that a genetic syndrome is present and is the cause of the individual's complaint (usually hearing loss) is not always received so favorably. Disbelief, denial, and anger are also common reactions to unwanted information. I believe there are several reasons for this. Some reasons apply to syndromes in general, but some are specific to the diagnosis of WS.

The first, and probably most compelling, reason patients deny the presence of a genetic syndrome results from the power of the word "syndrome." To most people, "syndrome" invariably means the presence of mental retardation, developmental delay, or cognition problems in general. Although mental retardation is not characteristic of WS, the word "syndrome" alone is enough to generate fear and to prevent the patient from accepting a syndrome-based diagnosis.

Another cause of disbelief results from family familiarity with and acceptance of the phenotypic features of WS. The family may "know" that family members have experienced profound unilateral deafness for four generations, but they also "know" that the deafness was caused by "normal" aging, or exposure to noise, or to measles in infancy. They "know" that blue eyes and prematurely gray hair run in their family, but they regard these anomalies as desirable family traits. Family members may be proud that they have "dad's blue eyes" or "aunt Sallie's white hair streak." They do not yet understand the relationship of these anomalies to the less desirable anomaly of hearing loss. No one has pointed out this relationship, and they do not have the scientific background to make that connection for themselves. As one parent put it, "I'd never heard of Waardenburg syndrome until my son was born. My parents were deaf and I grew up with facial differences and a severe hearing loss in my right ear. I never realized that I could pass deafness onto my children and I did not know that my hearing loss and facial anomalies had any sort of genetic cause."

In addition, individuals may ignore the phenotypic signs of WS because many of those features are regarded as attractive, even beautiful. Bright blue eyes, for example are considered very socially desirable facial features. The idea that beautiful features can indicate a syndrome is surprising to most individuals.

The opposite attitude is also possible. Perhaps the family phenotype is more unusual than attractive. Perhaps the presence of heterochromia, partial albinism, or prematurely gray hair subjected family members to peer ridicule. Perhaps family members feel shame at their "unique" appearance. In such cases, individuals may resort to hair dye, contact lenses, and makeup to conceal evidence of a genetic phenotype. The problem with this approach is that concealing the syndromic evidence makes it difficult to identify the cause of the patient's hearing loss. If the individual is unaware of the diagnostic significance of his or her physical appearance, he or she may be unable to provide health care professionals with important diagnostic information, and the health care professional may not be trained to ask for this information. In such cases, the relationship of syndrome to hearing loss may remain undiagnosed.

Finally, the words "genetic syndrome" imply that someone is at fault for the presence of the problem, in this case hearing loss. Although family members may logically know that the parents did not deliberately choose to have a child with WS, and although WS may arise in any child as a new mutation, there is still an element of blame attached to the parent whose genetic makeup caused the condition. The family may experience denial, guilt, shame, anger, or other emotions regarding the birth of a child with a genetic disorder. Helping family members cope with these emotions is challenging, and is often best done by someone with special skills in counseling. Chapter 6 details options for counseling individuals with WS and their family members.

Although as health care professionals, we may be unable to alter the attitudes of individuals toward their genetic makeup, we can alter *our* attitudes. The first step is to become aware of genetic problems through initial observations and then to subject these initial observations to formal diagnostic testing procedures.

Sometimes it is not the patient, but the health care professional, who hinders the diagnosis of a genetic problem. We may mistakenly believe that, unless we are physicians, geneticists, or genetic counselors, we have no business preparing family pedigrees or discussing genetic issues with family members.

It is true that issues such as blood typing, DNA testing, and other specific genetic treatment options are best left to experts with extensive training in genetics and genetic counseling. On the other hand, as medical care providers, we are all obligated to reveal our findings to patients, convey our concern and our reasons for concern, and to suggest short- and long-term plans of care for our patients. We are, in fact, legally liable for what we *do not* tell patients. Audiologists, for example, have been subjected to litigation for *not* informing the parents of children with genetically induced hearing losses that the probable cause of their children's hearing loss was genetic. If genetic problems appear to exist, the affected individual, as well as immediate family members, have a right to know that genetics may be the cause of their physical problems.

Patients initially consult health care providers for diagnosis of a problem. Perhaps they want to know how well they see or hear. Perhaps they or their children are having learning problems or difficulty achieving scholastically. What should we do when we suspect those problems have a genetic cause, but have no proof of this? For example, suppose a parent brings a child to your facility for hearing testing. In preliminary observations you notice that the child has bright blue eyes and a central white streak of hair in her forehead. The child's pure tone audiogram indicates a moderate bilateral sensorineural hearing loss. You notice that the child's parent has unusual facial features consistent with WS1. What should you do next? Here are general guidelines for resolving such issues:

- Ask for more information. Be specific to the issues that concern you. For example, you might ask, "Who else in your family has eyes like Beverly's? Does hearing loss run in your family?"

- Be prepared to tell the parents or the individual why you are asking these questions. Although you may understand the relationship between hair and eye color and hearing loss, they may see no relationship between the two and consider your questions irrelevant and intrusive. You might say, "People with gray hair, blue eyes, and hearing loss often have an inherited form of hearing problem called 'Waardenburg syndrome.' I am concerned that Beverly's hearing loss may be caused by a genetic problem. That's why I am asking for information about her physical appearance."

- Conduct or recommend additional appropriate testing to confirm your findings. For example, the presence of a WS1 phenotype coupled with the indication of sensorineural hearing loss on Beverly's audiogram justifies recommending speech audiometry testing and otoacoustic emissions testing. Recommend additional testing if it will help lead to a diagnosis of a genetic problem and/or if it will help you plan a solution to the patient's problems.

- Approach the possibility of a genetic problem directly. Say something like, "I am concerned that Beverly may have an inherited form of hearing loss (or whatever problem you are examining Beverly for). The reasons I believe this are that Beverly has blue eyes, a white streak in her hair, and a sensorineural hearing loss. This combination of problems often occurs in individuals with a syndrome called 'Waardenburg syndrome.' If Beverly does have this syndrome, other members of your family may be at risk for hearing loss. I would like to talk with you and your family about this. We may need to test your entire family for hearing loss. You may have questions about genetics that I am not able to answer. That's why I would like you to consider talking with a genetic counselor. Let's plan another meeting to talk about what we can do for Beverly's hearing loss, and how we can prevent hearing loss in your family." We are assuming of course, that the family wants to prevent hearing loss. Some families who belong to the Deaf community may consider hearing loss to be normal and desirable. Even if this is the case, the family is entitled to learn all the options for dealing with genetic syndromes.

- Document your findings in writing, and back them up with photographs of the patient. This is good clinical practice and provides you with visual support for your recommendations and your written reports to parents and/or affected individuals. Photographs are especially useful in determining family phenotype, as discussed below. If you believe a genetic problem is the cause of your patient's symptoms, begin by observing the patient's phenotype.

DIAGNOSING WS PHENOTYPE

Previous chapters discussed the major and minor phenotypic manifestations of all four types of WS in detail. Suppose a patient in your caseload appears to have a phenotype consistent with WS. What should you do to confirm that the problem really is WS and not a genetic syndrome with similar phenotypic features? The simplest and most cost-effective method is to conduct a thorough physical observation of the patient's face, take a careful case history, and develop a family pedigree. This approach has several advantages: it can be completed in a timely and cost-effective manner; is usually nonthreatening to the patient; is noninvasive; and can be conducted without using expensive specialized diagnostic equipment. The disadvantages are that this method provides physical evidence suggesting presence of WS, but cannot reliably diagnose the specific type. Sometimes this method provides evidence of pigment-disorder syndromes that are similar to WS. At best, this method provides the evidence needed to make appropriate referrals for genetic counseling, and genetic testing. It is also a good starting point for planning for specific therapies including speech therapy and aural rehabilitation. I recommend beginning observations with an overall observation of the patient's facial features.

Facial Observations

I find it most helpful to observe the patient's face from several vantage points: full face, both profiles, back of the head and neck, and top of the head. I also photograph the patient from these vantage points so that I have a visual record of my observations to supplement my written observations. I begin by examining the patient from a full-face perspective.

Full-Face Observation

From a full-face perspective one can determine facial *proportions,* facial *size,* and facial *symmetry.* Figure 4–1A shows normal adult facial proportions.

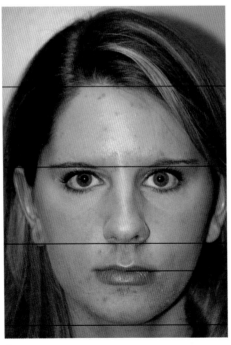 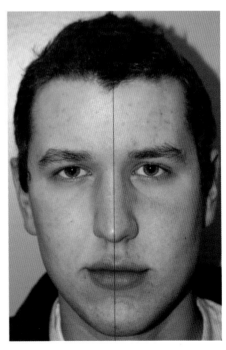

A.   **B.**

FIGURE 4–1. Normal facial proportions for adults.

Normally proportioned adult faces can be divided into three equal sections, as demonstrated in Figure 4–1A. These proportions are consistent for gender and race, but not for age. The faces of babies and small children are still growing, and their facial structures have not yet achieved their final relationships. Older adults may experience bone loss related to long-term use of dentures, and their faces may have undergone skeletal changes that affect their facial proportions. Individuals with WS 1 may also fail to meet these proportional guidelines because of the presence of dystopia canthorum and because facial asymmetry is common in individuals with WS. Facial *symmetry* means that both the right and left sides of the face are approximately the same size and shape. Many normal individuals, as well as individuals with WS of any type, may have noticeable facial asymmetry. The man in Figure 4–1B has noticeable facial asymmetry. The human nose is often asymmetric as a result of trauma. Full-face observations also allow observation of eye position, eye color, eyebrow appearance, structure of the nasal bridge, and hair color.

Eye Measurements

Physicians, geneticists, and genetic counselors often measure eye *position* to determine if the patient's eyes are at a normal distance from one another. The "normal" distance between eyes is approximately the distance of the length of one eye measured from corner to corner. Epicanthal folds can make normal eyes appear to be farther apart than normal. Geneticists and genetic counselors usually perform the W index and other biometric indexes to determine presence of dystopia canthorum. If you are not confident in your ability to accurately make biometric measurements, you can recommend that this be done by another medical professional if your initial visual examination indicates that such measurements are necessary.

Eye Color

Bright blue eyes are common in persons with WS. They are also common in normal individuals, so this feature alone is not compelling enough to render an accurate diagnosis. Nevertheless, blue eyes are often associated with syndromes in general and deserve a second look. Observe the eyes for heterochromia iridis, strabismus, and size and location of pupils. In some patients with WS, eye color may have changed from solid blue to patchy blue-brown during adolescence. Question the patient about eye color changes and ask if vision problems or cataracts are present. The eye problems associated with WS are usually structural, not functional, although there are reports of anophthalmia, strabismus, and amblyopia in specific populations of individuals. Remember that eye color can be concealed or changed if the patient is wearing contact lenses. Ask the patient to remove contacts while eye observation takes place.

Nasal Bridge Appearance

Individuals with WS 1 usually have a broad, flattened nasal bridge, sometimes with eyebrows meeting at midline. Epicanthal folds are often present because the flattened nasal bridge allows overlying skin to drape down over the inner corners of the eye. Because this condition is often more pronounced in infancy and childhood, I often ask adult patients to bring photographs of themselves as infants or children.

Hair

Observe the individual's head and facial hair for signs of prematurely gray or white areas. The classic position for white hair is just above the forehead. However, depigmented hair may be found in eyebrows, eyelashes, beards, sideburns, and in any place on the head. Even if the hair appears uniformly colored, ask the patient if he or she changed hair color with dye. Ask the person if his or her hair turned gray prematurely (before the age of 30) or if prematurely gray hair "runs in the family."

Profiles

Profile observation supplies information about the patient's ears, mandibular structure, dental relationship, and hair color and placement. In WS, pigmentary anomalies and retrognathic mandible are common. Facial profiles may be orthognathic (perfect), retrognathic (receding chin), slightly retrognathic (normal for most Caucasians), or prognathic (protuberant chin). Figure 4-2 shows the profile of a young man with WS. His mandible is slightly retrognathic, and he has a profound unilateral hearing loss. Retrognathic profiles are common in individuals with WS of any type.

Observe the appearance of the outer ears. Look for the presence of preauricular pits or tags. Notice the placement of the auricles relative to the rest of the head and neck. Individuals with very retrognathic profiles sometimes have auricles that are rotated downward and backward toward the back of the neck.

Back of the Head

A posterior observation point allows for observation of a patient's skin, neck, and hair. Because skin and hair contain pigment, this location often reveals pigmentary anomalies associated with WS. Persons with WS may also have vascular anomalies such as port-wine stain (Figure 4-3), sometimes called strawberry nevus, located at the base of the neck. Observe the back of the

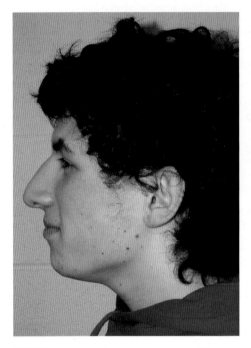

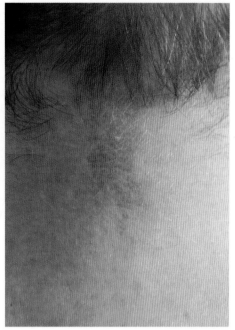

FIGURE 4–2. A young man with retrognathic profile and profound unilateral hearing loss. Notice that this individual also has numerous nevi on his jaw and neck.

FIGURE 4–3. Port-wine stain is a vascular anomaly often located on the back of the neck. This individual has a port-wine stain extending from the base of the neck, well into the skin of the scalp. Port-wine stains often fade or diminish in size over time.

neck for port-wine stains, freckles, moles, or depigmented areas of skin in otherwise normally pigmented skin. Observe the patient's hair for white or silver hair in otherwise dark hair, or for uniformly silver or very white hair.

Top of the Head

Observing the top of the patient's head is a good way to observe hair placement and color. It also provides a way to observe skull shape and symmetry. Observe the patient's hair for signs of WS as described above.

The presence of physical features of WS may strongly suggest the presence of a syndrome, but do not provide enough evidence for an accurate diagnosis, because several conditions have very similar phenotypes to that of WS. Differential diagnosis is sometimes required to separate these conditions from that of WS.

DIFFERENTIAL DIAGNOSIS OF WS

As observers, we must be careful not to reach inaccurate conclusions based on limited phenotypic assessment. Accurate syndrome identification depends on the presence of a *pattern* of anomalies, not on isolated unusual facial features. Several medical conditions have phenotypes similar to those of WS, and can be confused with it. These conditions usually involve pigmentary anomalies of hair, skin, and/or eyes. The following are brief descriptions of the most common conditions that can be mistaken for WS.

Conditions Causing Albinism or Partial Albinism

Albinism means lack of pigment in skin, hair, or eyes. A number of physical problems cause albinism, but not all of these problems result from genetic syndromes.

Nevus Anemicus

Nevus anemicus is a congenital deficiency of terminal blood vessels. The skin and tissue that should be supplied by these vessels may look pale and lighter colored than surrounding skin. This is a medical condition, not a syndrome, and it is not associated with pigmentary anomalies of the eyes or hair. Hearing loss is not present, nor are unusual facial features characteristic of this condition.

Hypomelanosis of Ito (Ito Syndrome)

This genetic condition occurs sporadically and produces symmetric depigmented streaks, patches, swirls, or sprays on the skin of affected individuals. These problems are present at birth and are sometimes accompanied by wide-set eyes and anomalous auricles. Skeletal anomalies have been reported in some cases. This is a comparatively rare disorder, with only 180 cases being reported as of 1992 (Wiedemann & Kunze, 1997). Hearing loss is not present in patients who have this disorder. The condition has been linked to an X/autosome translocation involving Xp11 (Hodgson et al., 1985).

Piebaldism

Piebaldism is an autosomal-dominant condition that has been traced to a mutation of gene 4q12–13. The phenotype of this condition is very similar to that of WS. Areas of depigmented skin frequently occur on the head and trunk, as well as in the eyebrows, eyelids, eyelashes, and forelock. Heterochromia iridis may be present. Deafness is not a characteristic of this syndrome, nor is broad nasal root or dystopia canthorum. Piebaldism is often found in patients of African ancestry. It is impossible to differentiate piebaldism from WS on phenotypic appearance alone. Case history information about family occurrence of hearing loss may be helpful in making the distinction, but genetic analysis is the only certain way of distinguishing between the two conditions (Baraitser & Winter, 1996; Wiedemann & Kunze, 1997).

Oculocutaneous Albinism/Ocular Albinism

Oculocutaneous albinism produces total absence of pigment in all of the individual's skin, hair, and eyes. If pigment is lacking only in the eyes the condition is called ocular albinism. The patient often experiences photophobia, strabismus, and low vision. Some patients have nystagmus (involuntary oscillation of the eyeballs). For most patients, ocular albinism is an X-linked type called Nettleship-Falls ocular albinism. This means that the gene that causes ocular albinism is located on the X chromosome and is passed from mother to son. A less common, autosomal recessive form of ocular albinism results from a mutation of genes 11q14–q21, and affects males and females equally.

Oculocutaneous albinism Type 2 has similar phenotypic features, except that skin and hair have a generalized decreased pigmentation and are pale, rather than white. Type 2 originates from a problem with the 15q11–q13 gene locus. Oculocutaneous albinism may be present in WS2, but genetic testing is needed for accurate differential diagnosis, because oculocutaneous albinism occurs in several other syndromes.

The National Organization of Albinism and Hypopigmentation (NOAH) provides information and support to individuals who have pigmentary conditions. The Web site also contains photographs of individuals with albinism, as well as information on annual conventions and educational presentations. For more information on albinism, see http://www.albinism.org or write the organization at: P.O. Box 959, East Hampstead, NH 03826-0959.

Vitiligo

Vitiligo is an autoimmune disorder that has been associated with mutations on chromosomes 1, 7, 8, and 4. Depigmented patches of skin are common on the face, hands, feet, elbows, knees, and chest. Hair may lose pigment, and the depigmented areas of skin may increase in size. Hearing loss and craniofacial anomalies do not accompany this problem. Some cases of vitiligo appear to be hereditary; others are associated with trauma, hyperthyroidism, diabetes, and adrenal problems. The main problems associated with vitiligo are cosmetic, especially when the condition occurs in individuals with very dark skin. Sometimes this condition resolves spontaneously (Simon & Janner, 1998). The following resources can provide support services and information about vitiligo.

American Vitiligo Research Foundation
P.O. Box 7540
Clearwater, FL 33758
Phone: 727-461-3899
Fax: 727-461-4796
E-mail: vitiligo@avrf.org
Web site: http://www.avrf.org

National Vitiligo Foundation
611 S. Fleishel Ave
Tyler, TX 75701
Phone: 903-531-0074
Fax: 903-525-1234
E-mail: vitiligo@billistic.com
Web site: http://www.vitiligofoundation.org

Conditions Producing Heterochromia Iridis

Heterochromia iridis occurs as an occasional anomaly in a number of syndromes, including Horner's syndrome and piebaldism (discussed above). The condition may also be associated with disease and trauma.

Horner Syndrome

Horner's is not a genetic syndrome, but rather a collection of symptoms that may be caused by a variety of etiologies. If the problems causing Horner's syndrome are congenital, the child may be born with heterochromia iridis, as well as one or more of the following symptoms: absence of sweating on the same side as the brain injury, paralysis of sympathetic nerve supply to the eyelid producing lid ptosis (drooping), and unequal pupil size. Horner's syndrome is symptomatic of a variety of neurologic problems including Arnold-Chiari malformation, brain tumors, meningitis, spinal cord injury, and Hodgkin's disease. It is not associated with hearing loss or additional pigmentation anomalies.

Eye Trauma

Eye trauma may destroy the pigment layer of the iris and lead to formation of scar tissue. Figure 4–4 shows the eye of a man who experienced eye trauma as a child when someone snapped a suspender fastener in his eye. He is legally blind in this eye. A close look at the injured eye (right eye in the photograph) shows bands of scar tissue across the underlying blue pigment that remains in the iris. This man's uninjured eye is brown and has normal vision. This is an example of heterochromia iridis resulting from trauma. Sometimes

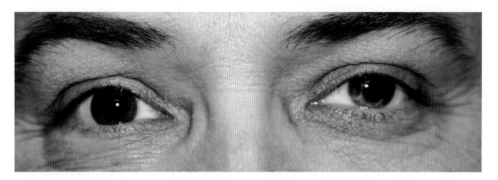

FIGURE 4–4. Eye trauma can sometimes approximate the appearance of heterochromia iridis. The eye on the left has lost brown pigment because of a traumatic accident in this man's childhood. His normal eye is brown.

this condition causes eye pain when the eye is exposed to strong sunlight. Corrective surgery or protective contact lenses may be needed to treat the problem. Patients remember eye trauma. Always ask the patient about the cause of an anomaly before assuming that it is genetic.

References for Differential Diagnosis

These textbooks are especially useful in making a differential diagnosis. The books are expensive, but are worth the expense if you work with patients who have genetic problems. For occasional use, interlibrary loan is an affordable option.

- Baraitser, M., & Winter, R. M. (1996) *Color atlas of congenital malformation syndromes.* London: Mosby-Wolfe. This atlas provides color photos of most major genetic syndromes, but does not provide extensive information about natural history or treatment of the problems caused by the syndromes.

- Jones, K. L. (1997) *Smith's recognizable patterns of human malformation.* Philadelphia: W.B. Saunders Co. This text is my personal favorite for comparing syndromes. In addition to descriptions and black and white photographs of major syndromes, the text contains comprehensive comparative charts of embryonic development and black and white line drawings of chromosomal anomalies. The book includes chapters on problem solving, morphogenesis and dysmorphogenesis, and minor anomalies. Normal growth charts are included, as well as a very useful appendix listing syndromes based on location of problem. For example, there are lists of syndromes with heart anomalies, syndromes with broad nasal bridge, microglossia, and the like. The size of this book is easy to handle, and it is not heavy, except in the intellectual sense.

■ Roy, F. H. (1997). *Ocular differential diagnosis.* Baltimore: Williams and Wilkins. Although this is a very specialized text for diagnosing eye anomalies it has excellent descriptions and comparative charts. However, it has no photographs, is diagnostic only, and contains no material regarding treatment or outcome of the problem. It is available in paperback.

■ Schneider, V., & Cabrere-Meza, G. (1998). *Rudolph's brief atlas of the newborn.* London: B. C. Decker Inc. Color photographs enhance written descriptions of most major problems of the newborn infant. The atlas includes topics such as deformations, chromosomal disorders, neonatal dermatology, and endocrine and metabolic disorders. Tips for differential diagnosis are included, along with probable outcome. This is an excellent all-round resource guide to the problems of newborn infants.

■ Simon, C., & Janner, M. (1998). *Color atlas of pediatric diseases with differential diagnosis.* New York: International Thompson Publishing. Like the preceding atlas, this one includes differential diagnosis of diseases throughout childhood. The color photographs are excellent, although the book is rather large and unwieldy to handle.

■ Wiedemann, H. R., & Kunze, J. (1997). *Clinical syndromes.* London: Mosby-Wolfe. This atlas weighs about 5 pounds, but is packed with black and white photographs of most major syndromes, including some European syndromes that are uncommon in North America. It contains comments about main and supplementary signs, etiology, prognosis, differential diagnosis, and treatment.

■ Zatouroff, M. (1996). *Diagnosis in color. Physical signs in general medicine (*2nd ed.*).* London: Mosby-Wolfe. The color photographs and descriptions in this text are organized by body part, with the section on the head being particularly useful. Most descriptions are of adult patients. The atlas has ethnically diverse descriptions and photographs. It is lightweight, and small enough to be easily portable.

FAMILY CASE HISTORY AND FAMILY PEDIGREE

Physical observations can be enhanced by careful discussions with family members, and by compiling a family pedigree.

Taking a Case History

If initial visual observations indicate a syndromic phenotype, I prefer to schedule a second interview with the family to discuss family history in depth. I begin by telling the patient or the family *why* I want additional family information. Although I understand the relationships between hair and eye color and hearing loss, the family may see no relationship and may consider such questions irrelevant. For example, I might say, "People with gray hair, blue eyes, and hearing loss often have an inherited form of hearing problem called 'Waardenburg syndrome.' I am concerned that your hearing loss may be caused by a genetic problem. That is why I am asking for more information about your family's physical appearance." I also give the patient a list of questions that I am likely to ask, so that he or she can discuss the questions with other family members or get the answer from family records. Scheduling a second interview has several advantages: it allows the patient time to adjust to the idea that a syndrome might be present in his or her family, it lets the patient gather materials and photographs that will be useful during the interview, and it allows the family members time to discuss family appearance among themselves.

I ask that patients bring photos of themselves as an infant and as a child; photos of family members that demonstrate signs of WS; as well as dates of birth, causes of death, and unusual facts about family members. I ask the patient to "draw a family tree" indicating birth anomalies, stillbirths, and marriages with close family members, and I ask that they identify the ethnic background of family members. I ask them to bring their family tree with them to the interview. This saves time during the interview itself, and opens the door for discussion during the interview.

Examples of genetic case history forms can be found in numerous textbooks. Some very useful examples include those provided by Milunksy (2001), Jorde, Carey, and White (1995), Peterson-Falzone, Hardin-Jones, and Karnell (2001), and Shprintzen (1997). A family history for someone suspected of having a genetically based disorder consists of basically two parts: general information that might indicate a genetic component and specific information that might indicate the specific problem under consideration—in this case WS.

General Information

General information, in this instance, does not refer to identifying material such as name, age, and birthplace. Rather, it refers to questions whose answers might lead to the likelihood that a genetic problem is present. I usually combine the interview with the taking of a pedigree (discussed below). Sometimes the patient has already constructed a pedigree. In that case, I combine the interview with discussions, and possible corrections, of the pedigree. Table 4–1 lists general questions that may produce answers indicating a genetic risk factor.

Taking a Pedigree

In the past, genetic counselors and geneticists were the professionals who constructed pedigrees. They still do this, but other professionals have begun using pedigrees to make initial diagnostic decisions as well. Speech pathologists and audiologists in particular are beginning to use pedigrees more frequently for the purposes of obtaining genetic information, and also to help make decisions as to appropriate patient referral. Figure 4–5 shows basic symbols used to construct a pedigree. Other symbols may be devised to represent conditions not portrayed by this basic code. I usually interview the proband and construct the pedigree from most recent to most distant generations.

The person who is first diagnosed with a problem is called the proband. Unless the proband is a small child or is developmentally delayed, he or she is usually the person interviewed. Patients often ask me "how far back" they should go to obtain family history. The farther back, the better. As we learned in an earlier chapter, genetic counselors look for patterns of transmission that might indicate the type of inheritance pattern. Autosomal dominant transmission usually produces a vertical pattern of affected individuals, and the problem is usually present in every generation. Autosomal recessive problems often present with a horizontal pattern of transmission and appear in several

TABLE 4–1. General Information to Obtain from Patients Suspected of Having a Genetic Problem

---

1. Birth date, gender, and familial relationships of all known family members. This can be easily charted as a pedigree using standard pedigree symbols.

2. Ethnic background of family members.

3. Cause of death for deceased family members.

4. Number and cause of stillbirths and miscarriages.

5. Presence of family-related hearing loss.

6. Indication of consanguinity (mating between blood relatives).

7. Presence of diseases that "run in the family."

8. Presence of mental retardation, cognitive problems, or mental illness in members of the family.

9. Presence of family members with known chromosomal anomalies.

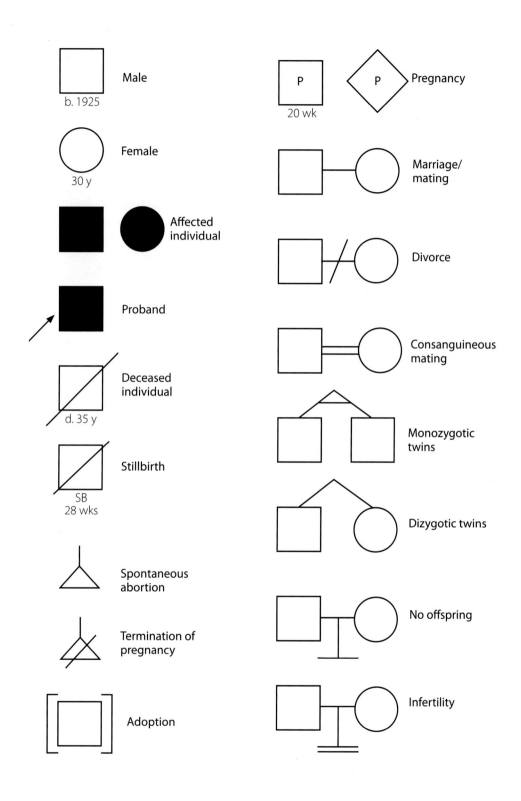

FIGURE 4–5. Symbols used to construct a family pedigree.

siblings within a family. Interviewing the family and constructing a pedigree is one way of discovering this pattern. As you talk with the proband or other family members, remind them that you want information about *all* family members, including those who have died before or at birth and those who have left the family through divorce or marital separation. Information about family members who have died stillborn or in infancy often provides some of the most valuable information when diagnosing genetic or chromosomal anomalies.

It is also helpful to ask family members about their racial and ethnic background. You can record this information above the entire family pedigree, or below the names and birthdates of specific individuals. Some syndromes are more common in some ethnic groups than others. WS, like many syndromes, is more common in consanguineous families than in others. Families who live, marry, and have children in small ethnic communities produce their children from a narrowed gene pool. The more closely the genetic relationships among individuals, the higher are the risks for individuals having genetic syndromes, including WS.

One of the disadvantages of taking a case history and constructing a pedigree is that the information you obtain may not be accurate or may have been sanitized by family members who want to conceal evidence of socially unacceptable behavior. Family members also vary in their observational powers and in their memory of pertinent facts. Discussing a family tree sometimes reveals startling or unwelcome information to the entire family. In one instance, I asked a student whom I suspected of having a genetic syndrome to construct a pedigree of her family. After interviewing family members, she told me that she had precipitated an argument among her aunts and uncles when she learned that one of her married uncles had not died of a heart attack as the family generally believed. Although he did die of a heart attack, he did so in bed with his 22-year-old secretary. Surviving family members were angered and scandalized when a grandparent revealed this information to the student. Other examples of information that can influence a family's accurate recollections of family history include instances of rape or incest, the (until now) unknown presence of illegitimate blood relatives in the extended family, the probability that a legal father is not actually the biological father, and adopted children who have never been told that they were not born to their adoptive parents. We depend on family members to provide truthful details about family relationships, but we cannot always be sure that the family will do so.

Specific Information

In addition to the general questions mentioned above, specific questions can often provide information indicating the presence of WS or, on the other hand, indicate the presence of syndromes that have phenotypes similar to WS. Table 4–2 lists specific questions that can help the examiner determine if WS is likely to be present in the family and if the family would benefit from genetic testing.

TABLE 4–2. Specific Questions to Ask Patients Suspected of Having WS

Ask the following questions, and follow up with discussions or probing for more information if the answers to the questions are positive. Ask for photographic documentation of affirmative answers.

1. Who in your family has prematurely gray hair? Does anyone have very white or silver colored hair?

2. Who in your family has patches of white hair on their head, eyelashes, eyebrows, or beard?

3. Who in your family has hearing loss? When did the hearing loss occur? What do you believe caused this hearing loss? What kind of hearing loss is it? Is it in one, or in both ears? Was the hearing loss sudden, or did it come on gradually? Does hearing loss "run in your family"?

4. Who in your family has bright blue eyes?

5. Who in your family has eyes of two different colors? For example, one brown eye and one blue eye, or both eyes that are partly brown and partly patchy blue.

6. Did anyone in your family have eyes that changed color during puberty?

7. Who in your family has oriental looking eyes? Does anyone ever say that a family member looks oriental, or has "crossed" eyes? Skip this question if the person you are interviewing is Asian.

8. Who in your family has eyebrows that are bushy, slanted, or that meet above their nose?

9. Who in your family has lots of moles or freckles?

10. Does anyone in your family have a small lower jaw?

11. Who in your family has port-wine stains or strawberry birthmarks?

12. Who in your family has patches of pale or very white skin anywhere on their body?

13. Does anyone in your family have severe headaches of unknown cause, or "migraine" headaches?

14. Has anyone in your family been diagnosed with ALS, multiple sclerosis, or a severe neurologic condition of unknown cause?

15. Has anyone in your family ever been born with cleft lip and/or cleft palate?

16. Has anyone in your family ever been born with spina bifida (open spine), anencephaly (no head), or other spinal cord defects?

17. Has anyone in your family had a spontaneously aborted or stillborn baby? What was the cause of the early death of this child?

18. Has anyone in your family ever been diagnosed with hydrocephalus?

19. Has anyone in your family ever had difficulty digesting food, especially as an infant or small child?

continues

TABLE 4–2. *continued*

---

20. Has anyone in your family ever been diagnosed with Hirschsprung's disease?

21. Has anyone in your family had upper arm weakness or upper arm anomalies?

22. Has anyone in your family been born with too many fingers or toes?

23. Has anyone in your family been born with crooked fingers or toes?

24. Has anyone in your family been born without eyes?

25. Did anyone in your family marry a close blood relative? For example, marriage between first cousins.

The most pertinent questions are those that help us identify family members who have genetic hearing loss. Again, there is room for inaccuracy because the family may have little information on the type, degree, or presence of hearing loss in family members of past generations. Even current family members with hearing loss may attribute their hearing loss to work-related causes or an illness in infancy, and not to a genetic cause, and they may in fact be correct in these assumptions. As you talk with the family, carefully observe the facial features of the family members. Remember that syndromes, including WS, sometimes arise as new mutations. The proband may be the first and only family member to have WS. Ask to see family photographs of previous generations of family members. Look for evidence of pigmentary anomalies in eyes, skin, and hair. If the photos are in black and white, ask questions about eye color and hair color. Observe photos of family members from both sides of the family because it is always possible, although unlikely, that members of both sides of the family carry the WS gene. This situation sometimes occurs in small populations where intermarriage from the same gene pool has occurred over generations. For this reason, I always ask the individuals what their ethnic background is. I have seen patients who are Turkish, patients who are of Northern Italian descent, and patients who are Welsh who have WS. In all instances the family were proud that they had maintained their ethnic identity by marrying only individuals from the same geographic location. In these cases, the family line remained ethnically "pure," but genetically flawed. Small gene pools allow for frequent transmission of undesirable genetic traits.

If time permits, photograph the proband and family members who are providing the family history. I document my findings in writing and add a summary to the written reports to the patient and to letters of referral. If what you see and learn from the family history and pedigree analysis leads you to believe that a genetic problem exists, you will likely be referring the patient for genetic testing and genetic counseling. The more evidence you can provide in the letters of referral, the more quickly and accurately the problem can be diagnosed.

AUDIOLOGIC TESTING

Because hearing loss is invisible and can occur at any time in the life of a patient with WS, it is wise to recommend taking a baseline audiologic assessment of all family members suspected of having the WS gene. A general audiologic assessment for any patient usually includes pure tone air and bone conduction testing, otoscopy (physical observation of the ear canal and tympanic membrane), and impedance testing to determine the mobility of the tympanic membrane and middle ear function. These basic tests are generally performed on every individual who wants baseline measures of hearing performance and ear health. Ideally, family members having, or suspected of having, hearing loss, should receive the additional battery of advanced audiologic tests described in chapter 5. These include speech audiometry and otoacoustic emissions (OAE) testing. Information from these tests is useful in differential diagnosis of hearing loss. Craniofacial teams often have geneticists and genetic counselors as part of the diagnostic team, but such teams do not always have audiologists available to do on-site testing. Some teams have audiologists, but do not have equipment to do advanced examinations such as otoacoustic emissions (OAE) testing. If your facility has a full-service audiology program, it is best to do the hearing testing as part of the initial diagnostic workup. If you plan to refer your patient to a craniofacial team, or genetic counselor, the results of the audiologic test battery can save the patient time and money in the long run.

Some programs, such as the Miami University Speech and Hearing Program, provide free hearing testing to WS patients as part of an ongoing research project. In other cases, patients may have to pay for audiologic testing out of pocket. Be sure to discuss this with patients before beginning costly and extensive audiologic testing.

GENETIC COUNSELING

If phenotypic observation, family history, and pedigree indicate the probability of WS (or of any other genetic syndrome), the family should be offered the opportunity to receive genetic counseling and genetic testing. Genetic counselors are specifically trained to compile family pedigrees, to make specific recommendations about genetic testing, to explain the results of genetic testing, and to predict the likelihood that a particular genetic problem will be transmitted to members of a future generation. They also determine the transmission pattern of the genetic condition and help formulate long-term treatment plans.

GENETIC TESTING

If the family wants to know if the WS gene is in their family, the most accurate way of determining this is through genetic testing. Even genetic testing may have limited accuracy for the rarer types of WS. WS genetic testing is done by sending a blood sample from family members to a laboratory where genetic analysis takes place. Although costs vary from one facility to another, patients can expect to pay from $1,500.00 to $2,500.00 for a genetic analysis. The recommendation for a genetic analysis usually must come from a physician, genetic counselor, or craniofacial team. Insurance companies vary in their policies regarding financial reimbursement of genetic testing.

SPEECH-LANGUAGE PATHOLOGY

Speech-language pathologists (SLPs) are often among the first health care professionals to treat someone with WS. Sometimes the patient does not yet know he has WS and has consulted an SLP for speech therapy for communication problems secondary to hearing loss. In this case, if the SLP recognizes the condition, he or she is obligated to make the appropriate referrals after following the procedures described earlier in this chapter.

Persons with WS often have normal speech and language skills. When WS-related communication problems occur, they are most often related to presence of hearing loss. Although cleft palate sometimes accompanies WS, most cleft palate repairs are completed before speech problems arise. The majority of early cleft palate repairs are successful, and few of these children ultimately need speech therapy. Children with WS and cleft palate are ideal candidates for team treatment. SLPs often plan early intervention therapy sessions for the infant in order to prevent the child from acquiring compensatory articulation errors and to encourage normal language acquisition and development.

Congenital sensorineural hearing losses can also prevent children from hearing and acquiring normal speech and language. Children who are severely or profoundly deaf must be identified early and fitted with appropriate amplification systems. Some families prefer that the child communicate in sign language and remain or become part of the Deaf community. Other parents of children who are congenitally deaf because of WS choose to enroll their children in programs or schools providing oral deaf education. Some children who are deaf are excellent candidates for cochlear implants. Remember that the type and extent of hearing loss must be determined before effective plans can be made to correct speech or language problems resulting from hearing loss. Parents, audiologists, and SLPs must work closely together to determine a long-term plan for treating both hearing loss and the communication problems resulting from the hearing loss.

All family members who have the WS gene should be identified, and all should at a minimum receive an audiologic assessment to establish a baseline hearing sample. Because WS hearing losses may theoretically occur at any time in the patient's life, and because congenital hearing losses due to WS may worsen at any time in the patient's life, hearing reassessments should be scheduled at least once a year. After WS-related problems have been identified, appropriate methods of treatment should be selected and implemented. Chapter 5 provides specific details on diagnosing and treating hearing loss in WS patients. Patients who have hearing loss plus additional physical problems, or patients who want to receive genetic testing and counseling as part of the treatment process, are often best treated by a craniofacial team.

CRANIOFACIAL TEAMS

Craniofacial teams are groups of health care professionals who specialize in treatment of anomalies of the head and face. Most large cities in the United States and Canada have craniofacial teams located in major hospitals. The American Cleft Palate Craniofacial Association publishes an annual ACPA Membership Team Directory. This directory lists team locations, specific contact information, and names and addresses of contact persons who are members of the ACPA. The ACPA also has a Web site for professionals and for individuals and families of individuals who have facial problems. Team treatment is an advantage for such persons because multiple problems can be evaluated and treated simultaneously in a central location. Other advantages to team treatment include demand for cost-effective health care services, interaction among health care specialists trained in different professions, and mandates of federal laws including Public Laws 93-112, 94-142, 99-457, 101-476, 101-336, and 105-14.

Craniofacial teams traditionally existed to manage the problems of children who were born with cleft lip and/or cleft palate. Recently, however, these teams have expanded their purpose and areas of specialization to treat children with multiple craniofacial anomalies, regardless of whether cleft palate is one of the anomalies. The professions represented on the team vary depending on the location of the team, the budget of the medical center where the team practices, the research interests or expertise of team members, and the availability of expert professionals to staff the team.

Teams may include any or all of the following professionals: oral-maxillo-facial surgeon, plastic and reconstructive surgeon, nurse, pediatrician, speech-language pathologist, pediatric dentist, orthodontist, prosthodontist, otolaryngologist, medical geneticist, clinical psychologist, social worker, genetic counselor, and, in some cases an audiologist. Most teams have a coordinator who interacts directly with the family by scheduling appointments, helping with financial concerns, counseling the family, and assisting family members with issues of transportation, follow-up, and initial interviews.

Team treatment is ideal for patients with WS who:

- Have cleft palate and WS

- Have multiple family members who are affected by WS

- Want to receive services in a central location

- Will benefit from multidisciplinary long-term treatment (as in WS 3 and 4)

- Require highly specialized surgery or medical treatment (cochlear implants, colon repair)

- Want plastic or reconstructive surgery to change their facial appearance

- Want to receive genetic counseling and family planning as part of their rehabilitation program.

In the above cases, craniofacial team treatment can save the patient time, money, and emotional stress by providing centrally located services from a team of highly trained professionals.

SUMMARY

This chapter has addressed the basic methods for differential diagnosis of WS. Chapter 5 will elaborate on diagnosis of hearing loss in individuals with WS.

REFERENCES

Baraitser, M., & Winter, R. M. (1996) *Color atlas of congenital malformation syndromes.* London: Mosby-Wolfe.

Hodgson, S. V., Neville, B., Jones, R. W. A., Fear, C., & Bobrow, M. (1985). Two cases of X/autosome translocation in females with incontinentia pigmenti. *Human Genetics, 71*, 231–234.

Jorde, L. B., Carey, J. C., & White, R. L. (1995). *Medical genetics.* St. Louis: Mosby.

Milunksy, A. (2001). *Your genetic destiny.* Cambridge: Perseus Books.

Peterson-Falzone, S. J., Hardin-Jones, M. A., & Karnell, M. P. (2001). *Cleft palate speech* (3rd. ed.). St. Louis: Mosby.

Shprintzen, R. J. (1997). *Genetics, syndromes, and communication disorders.* San Diego: Singular Publishing Group.

Simon, C., & Janner, M. (1998). *Color atlas of pediatric diseases with differential diagnosis.* New York: International Thompson Publishing.

Wiedemann, H. R., & Kunze, J. (1997). *Clinical syndromes.* London: Mosby-Wolfe.

CHAPTER 5

Audiologic Assessment and Treatment of Waardenburg Syndrome

KATHLEEN HUTCHINSON, Ph.D.

*T*his chapter describes a professional protocol for assessing hearing loss in individuals with WS. It also includes an overview of current treatment options, and illustrates assessment and treatment of hearing loss in four families with WS. After reading this chapter you should be able to:

■ List four specific audiometric tests that are appropriate for assessing WS patients.

■ Describe the types of audiograms you are likely to observe in patients with WS.

■ Compare the advantages and disadvantages of cochlear implants for patients with WS.

■ Name the type of hearing loss most often found in patients with WS.

■ List three possible etiologies for cochlear anomalies in patients with WS.

■ List three options for treatment of hearing loss in severe to profoundly hearing impaired individuals with WS.

■ Describe a protocol for family assessment and treatment of WS.

GENETIC HEARING LOSS

The auditory system is highly intricate, and many different genes are involved in its development and function (Arnos & Pandya, 2004). Scientists are still studying the formation of the inner ear from the time it is just a round opening called an *otocyst*, until it becomes a complex six-part ear that works with precision to allow hearing. Errors in inner ear formation may result from multiple genetic mutations. Approximately 1 out of 750 children sustain a significant sensory hearing loss prelingually, and an estimated 50% of these impairments have a simple genetic basis (Fortnum & Davis, 1997). Single gene mutations have also been demonstrated to cause late-onset hearing loss in adulthood in some families; acquired genetic hearing impairment in adulthood may be more common than we presently acknowledge (Steel, 1998).

Audiologists may be unaware of the phenotype for WS either through lack of experience treating patients with genetic syndromes producing hearing loss or because the patient has concealed the evidence of WS by dyeing his or her hair or wearing specially colored contact lenses. Patients with WS may confound the problem by reporting that their hearing loss originated from sources such as noise exposure or childhood illnesses. Hearing loss can be the only manifestation of WS with no externally visible indications of the syndrome.

SYNDROMIC HEARING LOSS

Genetic mutations can produce both syndromic and nonsyndromic type hearing losses. WS is a syndromic hearing loss and accounts for approximately 2% of cases of congenital deafness (Partington, 1964). Recent reports suggest that individuals with WS Type 1 have a 20 to 25% occurrence of hearing loss in one or both ears, whereas WS Type 2 has a 50% occurrence of deafness (Arnos & Pandya, 2004).

Hearing Loss Associated with WS

Hearing loss associated with WS can significantly affect the patient's quality of life and the development of speech and language. Etiologies of these losses include cochlear anomalies, cochlear defects resulting from developmental abnormalities such as hypoplasia of the cochlea, and auditory nerve fiber agenesis or absence of ganglion cells (Read & Newton, 1997). Rarey and Davis (1984) observed diminished numbers of spiral ganglion cells in the basal turns of the cochlea and atrophy of the organ of Corti and stria vascularis in WS 4.

Hearing patterns of patients with WS have both low- and high-frequency deficits, with some characterized by a U-shape audiogram (Liu, Newton &

Read, 1995). A bilateral symmetric sensorineural hearing loss is reportedly the most common type of hearing loss. The most frequent degree of hearing loss category was a hearing loss of more than 100 dB HL with no difference between WS I and WS 2.

AN AUDIOLOGIC ASSESSMENT PROTOCOL FOR TESTING PATIENTS WITH WS

As with all medical procedures, complete audiologic assessments require the integration of several key procedures. A case history including adequate information about the medical background of the individual must first be obtained. This documentation is important to both the current testing as well as any future evaluations.

The otoscopic examination ensures that the external ear and eardrum appear healthy. At this point, an immittance test should be administered to assess the motility of the eardrum. These procedures are usually well tolerated, and provide the audiologist with an opportunity to educate the patient about outer and middle ear anatomy. Figure 5–1 shows an adult patient undergoing an otoscopic examination. Once it is determined that the patient has a normal, healthy ear, further audiologic testing can begin.

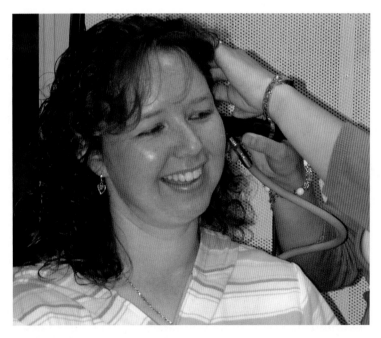

FIGURE 5–1. An adult patient undergoing visual examination of the tympanic membrane via otoscopy.

A pure tone test establishes hearing thresholds of the patient. After measuring these thresholds, the audiologist presents a series of words to the patient in an attempt to calculate his or her speech thresholds. The individual is instructed to repeat the words back to the audiologist exactly as they are heard. This speech recognition test differs from the typical hearing threshold test in that it provides a more adequate representation of the patient's ability to understand speech.

Otoacoustic emission testing is performed to assess the integrity of the inner ear. As tones are presented to the patient, measurements are calculated regarding the overall functioning of the cochlea. Although this evaluation cannot predict hearing loss on its own, its results contribute valuable information about the hearing acuity of the patient.

Final testing may include an auditory evoked potentials examination. This test may be an auditory brainstem response (ABR) or an auditory steady-state response (ASSR). Both examinations aim to measure the transmission of sound from the cochlea to the brain.

Case History

Before any audiologic evaluation begins, a case history form must be obtained from the patient. This questionnaire is composed of identification information, including home address, telephone number, and social security number. More specific information such as the reason for the visit, the assumed better ear, and the time at which hearing loss was first noticed are also included in the case history. Such data can explain potential causes of a patient's hearing loss.

The case history form for children is a bit more inclusive, possibly inquiring about the child's pre- and postnatal health. The child's speech and language abilities must also be recorded as a hearing loss could directly influence the development of these skills.

Although a case history form is essential to an audiologic evaluation, dialogue with the individual patient may be even more valuable. This interaction not only provides valuable insight into the communication abilities of the patient, but also supplies additional information not included in the written case history form.

Visual Assessment

Patients with WS, especially WS2, typically display different degrees of heterochromia iridis. Although usually normal, visual acuity should be evaluated by either an ophthalmologist or an optometrist. Both types of doctors examine and prescribe glasses, diagnose and treat eye diseases, and can evaluate how well a person uses their eyes together. Ophthalmologists are trained to do surgery whereas optometrists are educated in developmental aspects of vision such as behavioral and environmental factors. Behavioral assessment and interventions may be more beneficial to children with WS.

Specific Audiometric Tests

There are several fundamental hearing evaluations which the WS patient will undergo. These tests determine hearing thresholds to pure tones, hearing thresholds for speech, and overall functioning of the auditory nerve. Patients with WS often exhibit a sensorineural hearing loss that would be revealed by one of the following audiologic tests.

Otoscopy

Before any audiologic evaluation can be administered, an examination of the external ear must be performed. This procedure is performed with an *otoscope*, a handheld instrument that provides both magnification and illumination of the ear canal and tympanic membrane. Any excess cerumen present in the ear canal is then removed before beginning testing. This common procedure is performed on all patients and aids the audiologist in detection of any external ear malformations.

Acoustic Immittance Testing

Acoustic immittance measures impedance, or the opposition of sound at the eardrum. In a healthy ear, a sound wave will strike the eardrum and a portion of the signal will then be transmitted through the middle ear to the cochlea. The remaining portion of the wave should then be reflected back out the external canal. The energy of this reflected wave is most commonly measured by an impedance audiometry instrument. This calculation of acoustic immittance is a vital aspect of all hearing evaluations. The presence of middle ear fluid can be determined and possible audiometric findings may be predicted as a result of this examination.

Pure Tone Audiogram

During pure-tone testing, the patient is seated in a sound-treated booth and fitted with ear inserts or external earphones. When testing younger patients, visual reinforcement audiometry (VRA) is utilized to reward the child's auditory responses. With this technique, the child is rewarded with a visual reinforcer such as a light, picture, or animated toy. Figure 5–2 shows a child being fitted with an ear probe while seated on her mother's lap prior to pure tone testing. If a child is unable to tolerate insert earphones, sounds can be presented via a sound field through loudspeakers.

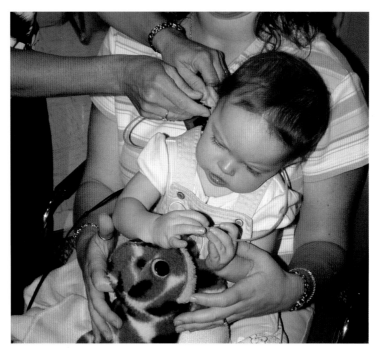

FIGURE 5–2. A young child is being fitted with insert earphones while seated on her mother's lap.

Pure tone audiometry is an evaluation that uses pure tones to measure a patient's hearing threshold at various frequencies. This assessment will reveal the softest threshold at which a patient can hear a pure tone 50% of the time. These results are then recorded on an audiogram, which serves to visually display the patient's hearing ability.

Speech Audiometry

Speech audiometry is often performed as a supplement to pure tone testing. Although pure tone thresholds provide information about the functioning of the auditory system, they provide little information about the patient's ability to hear and understand speech. Therefore, the stimulus used in this form of testing is human speech (as opposed to pure tones).

The most common testing materials used for speech threshold audiometry are spondee words. These words are composed of two syllables and are spoken with equal stress on each syllable. The patient is instructed to repeat each word back to the audiologist exactly as he or she hears it. The speech threshold evaluation measures the intensity at which an individual can identify speech sounds 50% of the time. This procedure is not only useful in determining the speech threshold, but also serves as an excellent check on the validity of the recorded pure tone averages.

A test of a patient's ability to follow or understand normal conversation is the speech recognition score (SRS). SRS can also be utilized to determine specific speech sounds understood by the patient. These tests of discrimination are performed in a manner similar to the speech threshold measures but at a constant intensity level.

Otoacoustic Emissions

Otoacoustic emissions (OAEs) measure the energy created by the outer hair cells of the cochlea. Their movement creates an "echo" wave that is transmitted outward through the middle ear and then detected in the ear canal with a sensitive, low-noise microphone. This evaluation is a quick and simple assessment of the integrity of the cochlea. Figure 5–3 shows an adult patient receiving OAE testing in a sound-treated facility. Although OAEs cannot be used to determine hearing thresholds, they are often able to detect hearing losses of 30 dB HL or above.

Two forms of OAEs can be administered. The transient OAE (TEOAE) presents a brief pulse of sound (known as a tone burst), and then measures the response between each presentation. In contrast, the distortion product OAE (DPOAE) utilizes two continuous tones of different frequencies. These

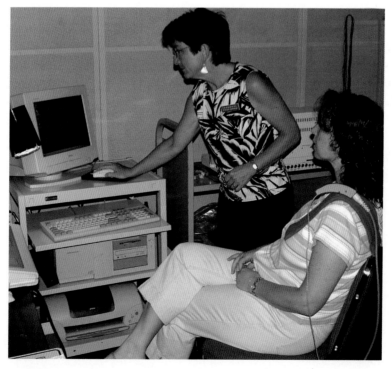

FIGURE 5–3. Otoacoustic emissions testing of an adult patient with WS.

tones are presented simultaneously and the patient's emission responses are then recorded.

The specific methods used to record evoked OAEs depend on the measurement unit and stimulus components. DPOAEs are one class of otoacoustic emissions that have been studied extensively in animal models. Liu and Newton (1997) found consistent patterns in DPOAEs in normal-hearing carriers of the genes for WS. In their study, all patients with WS type 2 had a "cookie-bite" notch between 1000 to 3000 Hz (a decrement in DPOAE amplitude). One-third of patients with WS type 1 had a similar pattern. These findings may underscore the fact that damage to the cochlea in WS is more common in type 2 than type 1.

Auditory Evoked Response Audiometry

Objective assessment of hearing also includes a category of measurements that detect the transmission of sound from the cochlea to the brain. Evoked responses measure the series of electrical changes generated within the cochlea to sound. The test most often encountered is the auditory brainstem response/brainstem auditory evoked response (ABR, BAER). Electrodes are placed on the patient's head and a series of clicks or tones are used to generate these electrical responses and estimate behavioral hearing thresholds. The ABR is used widely to detect childhood hearing loss, but its primary drawback is its lack of frequency specificity (Liu, Newton, & Read, 1995).

The auditory steady-state response (ASSR) is another form of auditory evoked potentials and has proven to be more useful in evaluation of hearing loss in children. Reduced test time and more reliable estimates of frequency-specific thresholds make this type of test more valuable than ABR testing (Werff & Brown, 2005). Additionally, ASSR can be used to measure hearing ability in a sound field with and without hearing aids.

Documentation and Report Writing, Privacy and Ethical Issues

Adequate documentation of a patient's history and test results is essential to any audiologic evaluation. The clinician is responsible for properly recording the results of each examination in a timely manner. These findings are then mailed to the patient and to his or her primary caregiver. It is important for each individual to realize that his or her medical information is kept completely confidential. According to the Health Insurance Portability and Accountability Act (HIPAA) of 1996, certain measures must be addressed in all clinic documents to protect and ensure the confidentiality of all client health information (Clark & Martin, 2006). Most individuals today are familiar with HIPAA assurances when they check into a physician's office. However, should a patient be unaware of his or her privacy rights, the patient will be fully informed of the HIPAA policy on entering medical clinics.

Discussion with Family and/or Patient About Testing Results

On the completion of the audiologic examination, results must be explained to the patient and/or guardian. Initially, the basic type and degree of hearing loss should be explained to the patient using his or her audiogram. Because many patients may be confused as to the meaning behind this form, it is the responsibility of the audiologist to provide a quick overview of the data. This explanation might include a distinction between normal hearing and a profound hearing loss as illustrated on an audiogram. Once the results have been explained, the audiologist should attempt to solicit questions from the patient and answer them with adequate detail.

Some patients and parents of patients may exhibit anger, frustration, sadness, and even guilt on hearing the results of their audiologic examination. Health care professionals must utilize counseling techniques to lead and assist these individuals through such emotions.

Referral to Specialists: Craniofacial Team, Genetic Counselors

After testing, a patient may need to be referred to another type of specialist. This referral may be due to a variety of reasons including the need for further diagnoses or treatment. Speech-language pathologists, otologists, psychologists, genetic counselors, and educators may be included in further treatment of an individual. Individuals with WS may experience deficits in several areas that cannot be managed by any one professional. When necessary, the audiologist will send the audiologic report to the desired specialist. Per HIPAA, this report must include a release form authorized by the patient or guardian to ensure confidentiality.

OPTIONS FOR TREATMENT

After an individual is diagnosed with a hearing loss, there are several options available for treatment. Typically, hearing aids are considered as a means of amplifying certain speech sounds. However, in cases of severe hearing loss, the patient may wish to consider a cochlear implant. It is important to remember that each case differs and all available options must be discussed with each patient.

Hearing Amplification

The most common treatment of hearing loss is the selection of a hearing aid. The main goal of an aid is to restore the patient's hearing ability to as close to normal as possible. Research has shown that hearing acuity is less influenced by background noise when two hearing aids are worn (Kochkin & Kuk, 1997). Additionally, the sound source is localized more easily by binaural hearing aids.

Hearing aids come in a variety of sizes, shapes, and colors to best serve the patient's needs. Also, a variety of hearing aid types, including analog, digital, and analog/digital hybrids are currently being sold. This variety allows for an impressive level of satisfaction among hearing aid users.

Cochlear Implants

Each year thousands of deaf children are surgically implanted with cochlear implants. These devices use surgically implanted artificial electrodes to stimulate the auditory nerve, thus bypassing the damaged cochlca. This intervention approach is similar to that of hearing aids as both function to amend the problem of hearing loss. However, unlike a hearing aid, the cochlear implant option is more intricate and its implementation requires significantly more time and planning (Xu, Thompson, & Pfingst, 2005). Figure 5–4 shows a young child with WS who has received a cochlear implant.

After a patient has been fitted with a cochlear implant, he or she will enter into a lengthy course of rehabilitation. The individual must be trained to

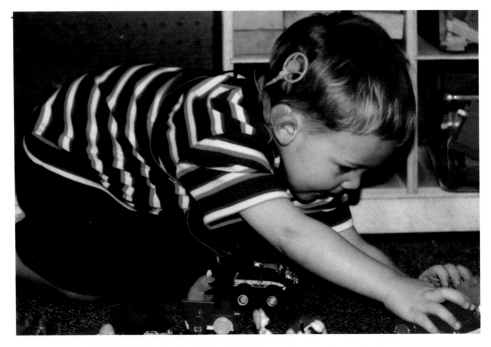

FIGURE 5–4. A child with WS and a cochlear implant.

recognize the unique sounds of the implant and discern recognizable speech from them. Although the head surgeon is initially responsible for interaction with the patient, a variety of other specialists may also be involved. If the patient is a child, teachers are often key components of this team.

Oral Education Versus Sign

Since the late 18th century, there have been debates about the proper mode of education for deaf individuals. The two main techniques that have remained at the forefront of this deliberation are oralism and manualism.

With the oral method, speech is emphasized as the individual is taught to read lips and rely solely on verbal communication. In contrast, proponents of sign language argue that manual communication is a more natural and efficient form of interaction among deaf individuals. Although the oralism/manualism debate continues today, the most logical solution is to educate each individual with the technique that best serves his or her needs.

Other Options

Some individuals with profound hearing loss may not be candidates for either hearing aids or cochlear implants. These individuals may need to be informed of a possible new role in Deaf culture. Entrance into Deaf culture requires association with other deaf individuals in the community. Members of the Deaf community primarily use sign language, although some use oral communication; members may have been born deaf or lost their hearing later in life. Individuals immersed in Deaf culture may not be interested in hearing testing, intervention, or genetic counseling. It is also not uncommon to have hearing members involved in Deaf culture. These individuals may simply be involved in the community in support of their family and friends.

IMPLEMENTING TREATMENT

Fifteen years ago the average age for a child to be diagnosed with a hearing loss was three years (Yoshinaga-Itano, 2004). Now, thanks to legislative mandates in 42 states requiring universal newborn hearing screenings, this age is steadily decreasing. Early intervention of a hearing loss is crucial in regard to implementing possible treatment approaches.

When planning intervention for a child with a hearing loss, several collaborative activities may ensue. There may be referral conferences including other specialists and recommendations for further medical and educational interventions. Interdisciplinary approaches involving a team of specialists will allow an individualized education plan (IEP) to be created suiting the child's individual needs; the IEP ensures educational opportunity for students with disabilities (Smith, 2000). The IEP is a quasicontractual agreement to guide, orchestrate, and document specially designed instruction for each student with a disability based on his or her unique academic, social, and behavioral needs. Design of an IEP will include a meeting with both parents and educators to assess the child's needs and current progress.

Reimbursement Issues

Patients with Waardenburg syndrome may exhibit all degrees of hearing loss. Some children and adults may not need any form of amplification but only guidance, hearing conservation, and monitoring. With more severe losses, individuals may require aural rehabilitation along with amplification.

For the child with WS and hearing impairment, early intervention programs are typically provided by county and state service programs. Specific service providers in audiology can address regional public funding sources. For adults, most insurance providers rarely include hearing aid purchases under their coverage. Professionals working with these individuals may be able to refer patients with WS to nontraditional funding sources for hearing aids and aural rehabilitation. Some programs such as the Sertoma Foundation, the Lions Club, and the Kiwanis organization may be willing to purchase or contribute to costs associated with amplification.

Reimbursement issues are very different for cochlear implantation. Individuals selected for cochlear implantation typically have specific criteria and a profound bilateral hearing loss. Many insurance companies treat implantation and follow-up intervention as medical procedures. Costs for the implantation device and surgery can exceed $50,000. Individuals in our clinic have switched employers to become eligible for cochlear implant reimbursement with another insurance provider.

Need for Long-Term Assessment and Reassessment of All Family Members

After a patient is diagnosed with a hearing loss, it is important to monitor his or her hearing acuity annually. An individual may find that his or her hearing is significantly worse than it once was, and this analysis is made from viewing past audiologic reports. Also, because hearing loss in patients with WS is inherited, a thorough evaluation of all family members is useful. This assessment can help explain the hearing loss or possibly predict future hearing loss and hearing loss in future generations.

Lack of accurate early diagnosis and treatment of WS-related hearing losses can significantly affect the individual's ability to acquire speech and language. Presentation of case studies illustrates the range of phenotypic variability in four families with WS and presents suggestions for optimizing diagnosis and treatment for patients at risk for WS.

SPECIFIC CASE STUDIES

Individuals with WS exhibit a range of phenotypic variability. This chapter illustrates this concept in four families; one family with WS 1, one with WS 2, and two with WS of unknown type. The case studies present suggestions for optimizing diagnosis and treatment for patients at risk for WS. Subjects with WS type 1 were selected from a family of individuals who represent the physical and clinical characteristics generally observed in such patients. Subjects with WS type 2 represent five individuals identified through genetic testing and three generations of affected and unaffected family members. The family members with WS2 described in this chapter emphasize the importance of interdisciplinary procedures for accurate identification and intervention. Two families described in this chapter represent subjects with probable WS of unknown phenotype; that is, they report family histories of hearing loss, pigmentation changes, and different colored eyes for four generations.

All subjects were examined otoscopically and all were evaluated to have normal tympanogram results. Cochlear integrity of all subjects was assessed using a Madsen Celesta 503 Cochlear Emission Analyzer to measure DPOAEs. Stimuli and recording parameters followed protocols established by Madsen Electronics (1994). DPOAEs were determined at frequencies 1000 to 6000 Hz to obtain a "DP-gram." Baseline pure tone thresholds were determined on a Madsen OB8-22 audiometer using insert earphones in the ears in a sound-treated room suitable for threshold testing (ANSI, 1991). The degree of hearing loss was determined by examining the values across the frequency range of 500 to 8000 Hz.

Family 1

The two Caucasian males with WS 1 in this study contacted our clinic after reading a newspaper article about WS. Subject 1 (S1) had recently had a son who had failed the newborn hearing-screening test in the hospital. S1 reported that he was diagnosed with WS as a teenager, initially observed with dystopia canthorum. S1 came to clinic with his wife and son (S2) for testing. S1 exhibited a mild low-frequency loss bilaterally and a U-shaped DPOAE pattern (Table 5-1). S2 was found to have a moderate to severe unilateral loss in

TABLE 5–1. Pure Tone Threshold in Decibels (dB) and Otoacoustic Emission Thresholds (OAE) at Selected Frequencies (in hertz) for the Right (RE) and Left (LE) Ears of Subjects with WS 1 and WS 2

	Pure Tone				Otoacoustic Emissions					
	500	1000	2000	4000 Hz	1000	1500	2000	3000	4000	6000 Hz
Family 1 WS1										
S1 Age 37										
RE	25	10	−5	5	10	9	3	−6	8	6
LE	30	10	0	5	9	5	6	9	11	5
S2 Age 1.5										
RE	45	85	NR	NR						
LE	25	25	25	25	15	9	11	5	16	23
Family 2 WS2										
S3 Age 73										
RE	0	5	5	10						
LE	10	10	10	15						
S4 Age 34										
RE	15	5	20	55	9	20	24	16	20	−4
LE	5	5	10	10	14	25	15	8	17	9
S5 Age 12										
RE	5	5	−5	0						
LE	5	5	−5	5						
S6 Age 10										
RE	95	105	100	105	NR	NR	NR	NR	NR	NR
LE	45	30	5	10	−7	5.1	5.1	0	14	6

RE = right ear, LE = left ear, NR = no response.

90

the right ear and normal hearing in the left; he was subsequently fitted with a hearing aid monaurally. S1's wife reports no history of hearing loss or evidence of WS. She recently contacted the clinic to report the birth of a second son, born with normal hearing and lacking the appearance of WS1.

Family 2

The four Caucasian family members with WS2 in the study were a mother (S3), her daughter (S4), and two grandchildren (S5, S6). Subject 3 reported that her husband exhibited normal hearing and died at 64 years of age from complications due to Parkinson's and coronary heart disease. All of her children show evidence of pigmentary changes, predominantly heterochromia iridis. S3 and S4 sustain normal hearing bilaterally. One female grandchild (S5) also displays normal hearing. S6 exhibits a profound hearing loss in the right ear and a moderate low-frequency hearing loss in the left ear (Figure 5–5). He chooses to wear amplification only in school. Table 5-1 displays the DPOAE results for two of the four family members.

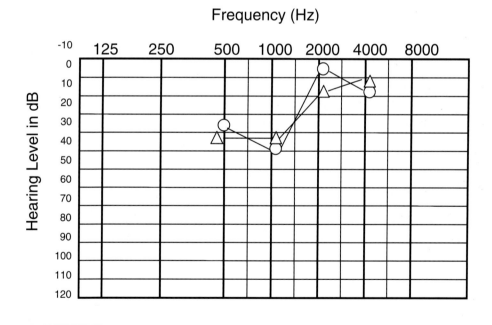

FIGURE 5–5. Characteristic low frequency audiogram associated with WS (S1 and left ear of S6).

Family 3

Five Caucasian family members (Family 3) with unknown WS type and phenotypic appearance suggestive of WS2 contacted our clinic after seeing an article written in the local newspaper. The participants consisted of a mother (S7) and her four children (S8, S9, S10, S11). Subject 7's husband exhibits no signs of hearing loss or WS and did not consent to participate in the hearing examinations, although he did provide case history information about his genetic background. Table 5-2 illustrates the age of each subject. S7 had normal hearing sensitivity with abnormal DPOAE results in both ears. S9 exhibited abnormal DPOAE at two frequencies in the left ear and normal hearing sensitivity. Subjects 8, 9, and 10 exhibited highest (best) values at 4000 Hz. All subjects except S7 had flaring eyebrows. Mild auricular anomalies such as prominent auricles, unusual shaped auricles, Darwin's tubercle, and low-set auricles were present to one degree or another in all subjects except S7. The most serious anomalies were not externally visible. These included missing kidneys and level 2 kidney reflux and profound sensorineural hearing loss. S11 had the most pronounced phenotypic manifestations of WS. These included congenital profound bilateral sensorineural hearing loss, blue eyes, hypertelorism, and dystopia canthorum (W index of 2.23). Kidney anomalies are not associated with WS. This family illustrates the possibility of more than one genetic problem for its family members.

Family 4

S12 was a mother who came to the clinic and subsequently brought in her son (S13), daughter (S14), and granddaughter (S15), all of unknown type with phenotypic appearances suggestive of WS 2. S12 was initially scheduled to be fitted for swim plugs and the audiologist noticed her retrognathic profile. S12 exhibited facial asymmetry and a profound hearing loss in the left ear with normal hearing in the right ear. S13, S14, and S15 displayed normal hearing bilaterally. S14 exhibited heterochromia and her daughter (S15) was born with six digits on each hand. DPOAE measurements for the four family members are displayed in Table 5–2.

PHENOTYPIC VARIABILITY IN WS

The four families just described illustrate the wide variability of phenotypic expression among family members and the unpredictability of the presence and degree of hearing loss in individuals with the WS gene. It also emphasizes the need for education of patients and medical professionals regarding early recognition and treatment of genetic syndromes in general and WS in particular.

TABLE 5–2. Pure Tone Threshold in Decibels (dB) and Otoacoustic Emission Thresholds at Selected Frequencies (in hertz) for the Right (RE) and Left (LE) Ears for Subjects with Probable WS of Unknown Type

	Pure Tone				Distortion Product Otoacoustic Emissions					
	500	1000	2000	4000 Hz	1000	1500	2000	3000	4000	6000 Hz
Family 3										
S7 Age 37										
RE	0	10	5	5 dB	–6	–22	–25	–21	–20	–17 dB
LE	5	5	10	5	–18	–28	–38	–25	–22	–20
S8 Age 12										
RE	5	5	–5	–10	10	0	–9	–9	15	16
LE	5	10	0	5	–18	–9	–5	1	10	–15
S9 Age 10										
RE	5	–5	–10	–5	–3	–6	–7	–4	7	–10
LE	0	0	–10	–10	–13	–7	–1	–13	0	–24
S10 Age 5										
RE	15	10	10	10	–12	–5	–8	1	–7	–11
LE	10	20	15	15	–5	–3	–1	–1	11	–11
S11 Age 3										
RE	100	95	NR	NR	NR	NR	NR	NR	NR	NR
LE	105	100	NR	NR	NR	NR	NR	NR	NR	NR

continues

TABLE 5–2. *continued*

		Pure Tone			Distortion Product Otoacoustic Emissions						
	500	1000	2000	4000 Hz	1000	1500	2000	3000	4000	6000 Hz	
Family 4											
S12 Age 59											
RE	5	0	10	10	5	3	–12.6	–10.1	3.9	–8.6	
LE	NR	NR	NR	NR	NR	NR	NR	NR	NR	NR	
S13 Age 39											
RE	10	5	0	10	–3.7	–.5	–2.5	–20.2	2.7	–1.5	
LE	15	10	5	10	–3.4	–8.5	–17.4	–10.7	–27	–1.6	
S14 Age 31											
RE	0	5	5	10	2.1	6.9	–4.6	5.9	17	1.6	
LE	10	10	10	15	6.4	5.8	8.3	–.4	15.4	7.9	
S15 Age 1.5 years											
SF	5	10	10	5							

RE = right ear, LE = left ear, SF = sound field, NR = no response.

The need for early diagnosis and treatment of hearing loss is of particular importance because hearing loss, if unrecognized and untreated, has long-term effects on speech and language acquisition. Finally, the experiences of these families illustrate the need for early, effective interdisciplinary treatment of the problems caused by the WS gene and for continued monitoring of hearing levels of all family members

The variability of expression of the WS gene in members of these families represents excellent examples of the ways in which phenotypic appearance can impact diagnosis and treatment of a syndrome. It is likely that the relatively mild expression of WS features in family members contributed to the delay in diagnosis and treatment. Socially penalizing facial features such as premature gray hair, large areas of depigmented skin, heterochromia iridis, or pronounced dystopia canthorum are usually recognized even by nonmedical professionals as significantly anomalous to warrant further examination. In all of these WS family members, however, facial appearance of all subjects, although mildly anomalous, was physically attractive. In addition, S7 chose to enhance her appearance by cosmetically altering her hair color and, in the process, eliminated a major diagnostic feature (white central streak of hair) from observation. For these reasons, only highly skilled observers were likely to suspect the presence of a genetic syndrome based solely on phenotypic appearance.

Recognition of WS

Early detection is especially critical when hearing loss is a component of a syndrome. Because hearing loss is invisible, and because the signs of hearing loss in infants are subtle, it is possible for this problem to pass unnoticed unless health care professionals are aware of the need to screen for it. S6's unilateral loss was not detected until he was screened in kindergarten. Neonatal screening, when available, is suggested for children with a family history of hereditary congenital hearing loss or for infants with syndromes known to include a sensorineural or conductive hearing loss. Three of these families had no previous history of congenital hearing loss, and the auricular and facial anomalies were mild. In any event, the hospital where the children were born had no system of neonatal hearing screening in place, nor did any of the various medical personnel involved in their health care recommend genetic counseling or hearing testing based on the children's physical appearance.

Kidney anomalies, although not a feature of WS, are sometimes indicative of syndromes with associated hearing loss. One might expect that genetic counseling and audiologic evaluation of S9 would have been recommended after he was discovered to have a missing kidney and unusually shaped auricles, but this did not occur. Only after the birth of S11, who was subsequently discovered to be profoundly deaf, was genetic counseling presented as an option.

One might also expect that the parents would have volunteered information about family history of renal anomalies or unusual facial features to health care professionals treating their family, but they did not. Although they were aware that there were physical anomalies on both sides of the family, they did not understand the implications of such anomalies. For the family with WS2, S3 remained unaware of the relationship between pigmentation changes and hearing loss until after the detection of hearing loss in S6. S3 believed that the "mottled" eye colors prevalent in her family were pretty, something that movie stars mimic with contact lenses. Only after genetic testing occurred did the family begin to share anxieties concerning future generations and understand the importance of monitoring the hearing level of all family members.

The lives of the persons in these families might have been changed significantly had the genetic background of their members been recognized before or at the time of the birth of the first child. On the other hand, as this study also demonstrates, the phenotypic expression of WS in any given family member could not have been predicted. According to S4, genetic counseling might have led her and her husband to make different choices in family planning and might have led to earlier detection of hearing loss in S6. Unfortunately, recognition of genetic syndromes requires awareness either by the person who has the syndrome or by the medical professionals who treat the person with the syndrome. Although multidisciplinary craniofacial teams are ideally designed for early recognition and remediation of syndromes such as WS, someone must refer the affected individuals to such a team.

Consistent Follow-up of Hearing Levels

Accurate monitoring of the hearing thresholds of all individuals with WS is critical to effective long-term care and quality of their lives and the lives of future generations. In this study, 11 of 15 individuals were found to have normal hearing (so far). However, it is uncertain whether the WS gene in individuals with normal pure tone levels has harmful effects on the inner ear.

Figure 5-6 demonstrates the obtained best ears' mean DPOAE results for all subjects with normal pure tone results. The normative data range is illustrated in the darkened area of the box for each frequency (Madsen Electronics). Responses below the lowest values of the boxes would be consistent with outer hair cell damage, usually consistent with hearing loss. On average, responses are within normal limits and do not suggest subclinical abnormalities. However, many individual responses fall below the normal frequency range from 1500 to 6000 Hz as shown in Table 5-2. Several individual subjects obtained DPOAE responses below −6 dB and still present normal pure tone results; these lower values are below the normative range obtained with this equipment. Individual findings represent a subclinical disorder involving outer hair cell function. The DPOAEs are inconsistent with a normal audio-

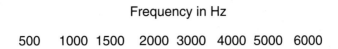

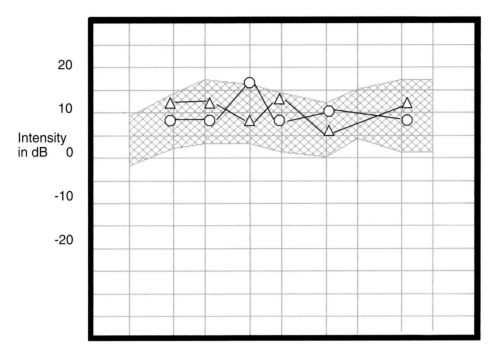

FIGURE 5–6. DPOAE-gram with average values of 11 subjects with WS who displayed normal hearing levels.

gram. This finding may depict an underlying disorder and suggests the possibility of future loss of pure tone sensitivity.

DPOAE results are consistent with S7's report of difficulty understanding speech in a background of noise. S7's hearing profile is also affected by her report of significant exposure to high noise levels without wearing ear protection. Distinguishing between hearing loss caused by noise exposure and hearing loss caused by WS complicates counseling for and treatment of subjects with potential future hearing problems (if any). Both the adults and children in this study have been advised to monitor hearing thresholds and DPOAE amplitudes as they mature.

Liu and Newton (1995) found normal pure tone hearing levels in a study of 26 patients with WS. On further testing using DPOAEs in a second group of subjects with WS, 7 of 8 patients were found to have lower amplitude DPOAEs compared to the control group (Liu & Newton, 1997). The authors concluded that pure tone testing might be insensitive to subclinical deviations occurring in normal hearing carriers of WS genes. However, 10% of the control group subjects also exhibited patterns similar to the WS patients. This finding reiterates the variability in expression of the WS gene and the difficulty in diagnosis.

SUMMARY

The case studies presented in this chapter reiterate the need for continuing interdisciplinary education of medical professionals regarding genetic syndromes, their early identification, and management. The WS gene affects the patient in a variety of ways. Many family members in our case studies were unaware that they had the gene because the expression of WS features was so mild. There is a great deal of variation in the sensorineural hearing loss among people with WS. At least half of those with the gene have no hearing problems. Only about one of five has a hearing loss severe enough to require some intervention to learn verbal communication. Some with the gene are totally deaf, and others are deaf in one ear, yet have completely normal hearing in the other ear. Regular follow-up for affected individuals with hearing loss is recommended to manage optimal treatment with hearing aids or other auditory devices, and to discuss possible treatment using a cochlear implant.

REFERENCES

American National Standards Institute. (1991). Maximum permissible ambient noise levels for audiometric test rooms (ANSI S3.1). New York: Author.

Arnos, K. S., & Pandya, A. (2004). Genes for deafness and the genetics program at Gallaudet University. In J. Vickrey Van Cleve (Ed.). *Genetics, disability, and deafness* (pp. 111–126). Washington, DC: Gallaudet University Press.

Clark, J., & Martin, F. (2006). *Introduction to audiology.* Austin, TX: Allyn and Bacon.

Fortnum, H., & Davis, A. (1997). Development of the vertebrate ear: Insight from knockouts and mutants. *Trends in Neurosciences, 22,* 263–269.

Kochkin, S., & Kuk, F. (1997).The binaural advantage: Evidence from subjective benefit and customer satisfaction data. *The Hearing Review, 4*(4), 29–34.

Liu, X. S., & Newton, V. E. (1995). Waardenburg syndrome type II: Phenotypic findings and diagnostic criteria. *American Journal of Medical Genetics, 55,* 95–100.

Liu, X. S., & Newton V. E. (1997). Distortion product emissions in normal-hearing and low-frequency hearing loss carriers of genes for Waardenburg syndrome. *Annals of Otorhinolaryngology, 106,* 220–225.

Liu, X. S., Newton V. E., & Read, A. P. (1995). Waardenburg syndrome type II: Phenotypic findings and diagnostic criteria. *American Journal of Medical Genetics, 55,* 95–100.

Madsen Electronics. (1994). *Celesta 503: Distortion Product Emissions Analyzer operation manual.* Coopenhagen, Denmark: Author.

Partington, M. W. (1964). Waardenburg syndrome and heterochromia iridum in a deaf school population. *Canadian Medical Association Journal, 90,* 1008–1017.

Rarey K. E., & Davis, L. E. (1984). Inner ear anomalies in Waardenburg syndrome associated with Hirschsprung's disease. *International Journal of Pediatric Otorhinolaryngology, 8,* 181–189.

Read A. P., & Newton, V. E. (1997). Waardenburg syndrome. *Journal of Medical Genetics, 34,* 656–665.

Smith, S. (2000). Creating useful Individualized education programs (IEPs). The Educational Resources Information Center Digest #E600. Available at: http://www.ldonline.org/ld_indepth/iep/ed449636.html.

Steel, K. P. (1998). A new era in the genetics of deafness. *New England Journal of Medicine, 339,* 1545–1547.

Werff, K. R., & Brown, C. J. (2005). Effect of audiometric configuration on threshold and suprathreshold auditory steady-state responses. *Ear and Hearing, 26*(3), 310–326.

Xu, L.,Thompson, C. S., & Pfingst, B. E. (2005). Relative contributions of spectral and temporal cues for phoneme recognition. *Journal of the Acoustical Society of America, 117*(5), 3255–3267.

Yoshinaga-Itano, C. (2004). Levels of evidence: universal newborn hearing screening (UNHS) and early hearing detection and intervention systems (EHDI). *Journal of Communication Disorders, 37*(5), 451–465.

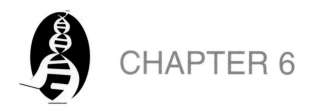

CHAPTER 6

Counseling Families with Waardenburg Syndrome-Related Hearing Loss

LAURA J. KELLY, Ph.D

*F*rom a parent's perspective, few experiences are more difficult than learning their child has a permanent hearing loss. In the case of families with Waardenburg (WS) syndrome, the process of informing family members of the presence of the hearing loss is often complicated by several factors. The diagnosis of the hearing loss may be the precursor to learning that the family as a whole has a genetic disorder. This information generates uncertainty of who else in the family may eventually be affected, and the knowledge that a progressive hearing loss could appear in present as well as future family members. This chapter explores the issues accompanying the diagnosis of a hearing loss caused by WS. After reading the chapter you will be able to:

■ List the steps used to inform a family of the diagnosis of WS-related hearing losses.

■ List the specific emotional responses that often follow the diagnosis of a hearing loss associated with WS.

■ Describe the different stages associated with grieving and ultimately accepting the presence of a hearing loss.

■ Describe a health care professional's appropriate responses to a patient's emotional states.

■ List the signs of significant emotional stress indicating that an individual may have unresolved grief.

PATIENT-CENTERED DIAGNOSIS

Informing an individual of the diagnosis of hearing loss is not just about providing facts and documentation of the existence of a disorder. Health care professionals have the responsibility of presenting the information in a manner that acknowledges that the information is potentially life-changing. It is especially important when informing parents that their child has a hearing loss. Health care professionals need to be sensitive to the chain of events they are about to trigger and develop the skills to present the diagnosis and provide appropriate support. Perhaps the process is best called "patient-centered diagnosis." It differs from the long-term diagnosis in that the label suggests the need for sensitivity to, as well as understanding of, facts during the potentially volatile and emotional interaction following the diagnostic session. The practice of respecting both the emotional and physical preferences of the patient is commonly referred to as "patient-centered care." The label is taken from "patient-centered therapy" coined by Carl Rogers (1951) to describe his theory of counseling, which suggested that an open and supportive relationship between the professional and the patient was crucial for effective care.

There are three possible scenarios a health care professional may encounter when diagnosing a hearing loss associated with Waardenburg's syndrome. The first involves testing a family with a known history of the syndrome. In the second scenario, the family may suspect the presence of Waardenburg but never has had genetic counseling to confirm it. In the third case, the person or family arrives for the hearing test and, as a result of the history, examination, and testing, the audiologist suspects an etiology of WS. Health care professionals should not assume that a family who has undergone genetic counseling is fully aware of the possibility that hearing loss exists as part of the syndrome. A survey of parents who had undergone genetic testing for deafness and hard-of-hearing conditions revealed that most respondents had a poor understanding of genetics (Brunger et al., 2000). There was little difference in understanding of hearing loss between the parents who had had genetic testing and parents who had not. More than one third of the parents surveyed who received genetic testing indicated their child did not carry the gene for hearing loss, or that future children would not be hearing impaired, when there was in fact potential for both to occur. We cannot be certain that patients are prepared for the news that their child has a hearing loss. All three possible scenarios should be handled as if the parent were unprepared to hear the news that their child has a hearing loss. In addition, in the case of a progressive hearing loss, the same care should be taken in informing caregivers of change in hearing level as when a caregiver is initially informed of the hearing loss. Although the caregiver may have intellectually accepted the possibility that his or her child's hearing levels could decline, the emotional response can be strong.

Setting

A six-step protocol has been proposed by Buckman (1992) to assist medical professionals who must deliver bad news to patients. A modified protocol for use in audiology settings is summarized in Table 6–1. The first step suggests that professionals create a setting appropriate to the task of delivering emotionally charged information. *Setting* refers to creating an environment that is as private and as comfortable as possible. When setting up the physical space, make provisions so that all parties are seated and the professional can make eye contact with the family. I have found an open seating arrangement without the barrier of a desk between the health care professional and the family works well. A table or desk positioned to the side allows me to have papers, tissues, or other items readily available for use during the counseling session.

Make arrangements to prevent intrusions from telephones (cell and office), pagers, and other staff members and allow sufficient time to interact with the caregivers. Kovarsky, Kurtzer-White, and Maxwell (2004) conducted focus groups to identify common themes experienced by parents who were informed their child had a possible hearing loss. One parent reported that the audiologist spent only 5 to 10 minutes discussing the results. In offices where pediatric testing is common, initiate procedures to allow more time for appointments that have the potential for lengthy post-test counseling. When the time allotted is insufficient, I suggest taking a few minutes to inform your next patient that there will be a delay because of time requirements of the preceding patient and offer the patient the opportunity to reschedule. When I do this myself, as opposed to relegating the task to office staff, I find that my patients are very accommodating, because they see I care enough about them

TABLE 6–1. Recommended Steps for Discussing a Diagnosis

1. Create an environment that is quiet, private, and comfortable.

2. Arrange sufficient time for the session.

3. Ask the caregiver their perceptions of the child's ability to hear at home and of the responses observed during testing.

4. Ask the caregiver how they want the information presented.

5. Present the test results with compassion in the manner requested by the caregiver. Link the results to the caregiver's observations of the child's behavior at home and/or during the test.

6. Address the caregiver's emotions with empathy, silence, and support.

7. Before the caregiver leaves, briefly summarize the results again and with the caregiver's help, devise a course of action for the short-term.

Source: Adapted from Buckman (1992)

to speak with them personally. In offices with more than one audiologist, a colleague may be able to see the next person.

If there is no possibility of extending the time available, inform the caregiver of the time constraints at the onset of the process and assure the patient or caregiver of your concern that they be fully informed. Near the end of the diagnostic session after providing initial information, remind the caregiver of the time constraints and end by arranging more time together in a subsequent session. Such arrangements should include ensuring that other family or friends are present. Even when sufficient time has been allotted, it may be necessary to schedule an additional appointment to allow full family participation. Additional appointments have the added advantage of permitting time for family members to further process the news and to provide an opportunity for other members to receive information that is not filtered through the emotional response of the caregiver who was present at the initial diagnosis. If an additional appointment is scheduled, it should be done within a day or two of the initial diagnosis.

Assessing Understanding

Once the family members are settled in an appropriate space, the health care professional should find out what the family understands about the testing process and how it relates to their own observations of their child's behavior. In the case of hearing testing, involve the family members as much as possible. Involvement might include handing the child toys during conditioned play audiometry, sitting in the booth with the audiologist and observing child behavior, or holding the child during behavioral observation audiometry. By participating, caregivers will have a better understanding of the testing and will also have seen the presence and absence of responses to the stimuli. They have a chance to compare what they are seeing with their own experiences. Asking the parent's perception of how the testing went enables the audiologist to note the parent's attitude toward the child's hearing loss and the audiologic testing process (Luterman, 2001).

Respecting Patient Preferences

The next step is an invitation for the patient and/or parents to share their preference for how the information is delivered (Buckman, 1992). Do they prefer a detailed accounting of each test and the conclusions, or do they prefer a summary? Asking the caregivers' preference provides the information necessary to alter diagnostic counseling to fit different personalities, is a gesture of respect, and provides the patient and parents with some control in a situation in which they may be feeling powerless. Some individuals want to know all the details from the beginning even if they were present during the testing.

The information places what they have seen in context and gives them time to collect their thoughts. Others will want to begin to discuss only the outcome of the tests. In many cases, parents have already come to the conclusion that their child has a hearing loss and the testing has confirmed their concerns.

Imparting Information

The invitation leads to providing the family with knowledge of the test results and reinforcing what the parents already know to be true. Some professionals suggest opening the knowledge stage with a statement that will prepare the family for bad news. Alternatives include: "I know the results today are not going to be what you hoped" (Buckman, 1992) or "I am sorry to have to confirm your suspicions that your child has a hearing loss."

Recent research suggests that using such phrasing may imply a negative professional judgment of syndromes and disabilities and, by association, the individual. A study by Skotko (2005a) indicates mothers were upset when physician's language suggested that the birth of their child, who had Down syndrome, was regrettable. Health care professionals should take care to avoid similar wording when talking with families with syndromes, and with families within the Deaf community. For those who view Deaf culture as part of their identity, implying that having a deaf child is regrettable can be very upsetting and seriously disrupt the professional/patient relationship. Professionals should consider using wording that confirms the presence of reduced hearing without impugning the child or the hearing loss. Keep in mind that at this point the parents may have difficulty separating their child as a person from his or her hearing ability or the syndrome. I therefore suggest phrasing such as, "the results today expand on your own observations. John does have a hearing loss that greatly affects what he hears." Notice the absence of "I am sorry" or "I regret," which suggests your judgment. If or when the client expresses feelings of loss and grief, you may indicate that you empathize with statements such as, "hearing your suspicions confirmed can be very hard." Also statements such as "I am sorry to be the one telling you this, but . . . " could be interpreted to mean your personal regret at having to share this time of grief with the family (e.g., I wish someone else could have done this for me and I don't want to be here or have to do it). Nonverbal signals may also convey inappropriate messages. Parents have reported that body language is very important (Skotko, 2005b). Failure to make eye contact was specifically cited by parents as an indication of the physician's negative attitude toward the child and the disability. Health professionals should develop the habit of monitoring their word choices and body language. Small changes in method of conveying "bad" news have the potential to make a big difference in the way parents respond to you.

Whether the patient prefers information in detail or as a summary, the audiologist should tie in parent's observations when presenting the results.

Statements such as, "You indicated when we first talked that Jane did not seem to respond to some sounds. As you could see during the tone test she showed the same lack of response here." Connecting the caregiver's everyday experiences with the test outcome helps place the test into a familiar context and reduces the "deniability" of the results (Luterman, 2001). It is more difficult to claim a test was wrong when the outcome agrees with what they have observed themselves. Use conversational language and avoid the use of professional jargon. Even if the individual is well educated, the initial shock of the results may make it difficult to follow a conversation after the news is imparted. Provide the facts in small cohesive groupings, pausing frequently for several seconds to allow time for processing, questions, and emotional responses. Be prepared for the need to repeat information and do not be surprised if few facts are retained upon return visits.

At this point in the diagnostic process, the caregiver may ask about the cause of the hearing loss. When the family history and the physical characteristics indicate that WS is a possibility the health care professional has the responsibility of making this information known. It is important to make clear that, although the markers are present, there is no way to be certain without genetic testing.

Providing Emotional Support

Being supportive and responsive to the emotions resulting from the diagnosis is perhaps the most important part of the counseling process. The range of emotions experienced by parents and caregivers are described in more detail in the next section. The immediate reaction will vary from person to person and sometimes with the degree of hearing loss identified. The caregiver may be quiet and unresponsive, cry, express disbelief, or become angry. Many professionals are uncomfortable when a patient expresses strong emotions, in part because they do not know how to respond. The single most valuable response is silence. Too often professionals feel the need to fill space with more information instead of letting individuals absorb the news they have just received. If the patient remains quiet for some minutes, an appropriate statement would be, "Can you share with me how you are feeling?" This statement gives the individual permission to talk about his or her emotions if he or she is concerned about expressing them.

A simple and effective way of showing your support is by repeating or paraphrasing what the caregiver has said. For example, if the caregiver says, "I can't believe this is happening, I was hoping it was something temporary like when he had an ear infection." The audiologist might respond with "The news is hard for you to accept."

I have found many audiology students are uncomfortable when they are first asked to practice using repetitive statements during training. They indicate that repeating back what someone has just said rather than responding with something new feels awkward. In addition, they think the patient will be frustrated and annoyed when someone "parrots" back their own words to them. After using repetitive statements, they report that the person with whom they interacted either did not notice they were using them, felt that the person was intent on understanding them, and/or expressed appreciation for the opportunity to talk about how they felt without someone offering personal opinions. The students also report that using repetition became less awkward over time to the extent that they find themselves using rephrasing in personal interactions to improve communication and understanding with friends and family.

Reflective responses take the concept of repetition a bit further by rephrasing the patient's statement to reflect the emotional content or other underlying meaning. Not all patients will state openly that they are angry, confused, or in pain. A reflective response to the statement, "I knew I should have followed my instincts sooner, maybe something could have been done to correct it," could be, "You feel guilty you did not get testing sooner." The difference between the two statement types can be very important. A caregiver needs to know the audiologist is listening for how he or she feels, not just the facts of the situation. A reflective response that addresses the emotion can be followed later by a content response that seeks to provide correct information.

Some student clinicians are concerned about making mistakes. "What if I am wrong about what the person is feeling?" A reflective statement provides the opportunity for the patient to correct your misperception and/or to expand on your comment so that you gain a better understanding and he or she feels supported. By preceding your reflective statement with phrases such as:

"I hear you saying that you feel . . . "

"I want to understand, you seem to be feeling . . . "

you signal the patient that you are interested and wish to be corrected if you are in error.

It is never appropriate to say "I understand what you are going through." This statement, more than any other, is likely to trigger anger and resentment from the caregiver. Although the audiologist may have an intellectual understanding of the emotional process or feel empathy because of experiencing similar life crises, the circumstances surrounding each family are different. The caregiver is experiencing an emotional pain that is unique at that moment in time and health care professionals should recognize and respect that situation. Clinicians should also avoid trivializing the caregiver's response by making statements such as "It is only a mild hearing loss" or "You should not be concerned, she or he can still hear most of the speech sounds." Although it is true that there are different degrees of hearing loss and the impact varies for each child, the caregiver needs time to process and accept the presence of the hearing loss. It is still a loss for them and a change in their perception of how the world will be for their child. Alternative statements that help provide support and appropriate optimism would be, "There are a number of ways I can provide you with help, during future visits we can go over them in detail. If you wish, I can also provide you with names of other parents to contact who have had similar experiences." It is also appropriate to help them understand that what they are feeling is normal. "Yes, it can be very confusing to try and absorb all of this information at once" or "You want to help your child, of course you feel sad."

Ending the Diagnostic Session

The final step in diagnostic counseling is to summarize the information that has been given and allow adequate time for questions. The questions will often focus on treatment options and can be used to work with the caregiver to form a plan of action. The plan may be very short-term and as simple as planning for further testing or setting up the next meeting with additional family members or friends. The decisions should reflect the desires of the caregiver and respect the fact that he or she may not be in a position to make long-term decisions. There are a variety of intervention options and the caregiver has a right to be given time to explore all of them.

Emotional support is just as important in subsequent appointments as it is during the initial diagnosis. Emotional responses will change over time and health care professionals should be alert to those changes. Of necessity, there will be an increase in the presentation of factual content. During follow-up appointments, the health care professional should review important material from the last meeting such as treatment options and have materials ready that contain educational resources and information about support systems (Clark & English, 2004). Any written materials should be checked to ensure a low level of readability and that professional jargon is limited and clearly defined. An attempt also should be made to document the nature of the information provided (Clark & English, 2004). It may be helpful to find out what resources for information and support the family is accessing on their own. Encourage them to keep their own records and to bring in any information they find confusing. In this way, the health care professional can ensure that caregivers have complete and accurate information to guide them in the decision-making process. Independent record keeping may also help the caregiver maintain a sense of control in chaotic times, become a long-term personalized resource, and help reduce dependence on the health care professional.

THE GRIEF PROCESS

With the advent of newborn hearing screening, it is becoming far more likely that infants with congenital hearing losses will be identified shortly after birth. Confirmation that a child has a hearing loss can trigger many emotions.

It is not uncommon for parents to enter into a cycle of grieving similar to that of a person who experiences a death in the family. The presence of a hearing loss and/or a syndrome represents the death of the ideal child. The model of grieving that is most often cited was first proposed by Kubler-Ross in 1969. The stages she identified include denial, anger, bargaining, depression, and acceptance. Other models have been proposed specifically for parents who are coping with the diagnosis of a chronic illness, syndrome, or disorder. After many years of working with parents of children with hearing loss, Luterman (2001) suggested that the four states of denial, resistance, affirmation, and integration are common.

He is quick to point out, however, that there are many emotions associated with the states and that the process is not linear. The behaviors and emotions associated with the state may overlap and/or parents may revisit the state's concomitant emotions at different times in the child's life. In the case of hearing loss associated with WS, the parents may have to deal with the grieving process repeatedly if the child's hearing loss is progressive.

Denial

A common scenario following the diagnosis of the hearing loss includes initial disbelief of the diagnosis. The disbelief may manifest itself by a period of inaction in which the parents fail to follow through on recommendations. They may seem unable to make decisions regarding their child, themselves, or other members of the family. Another common reaction is to seek additional testing from a series of different professionals in the hope that one or more will contradict the initial findings. Seeking a second opinion should not be automatically assumed to be "diagnosis shopping." Seeking additional professional advice from professionals with extensive experience with the population or disorder is often a wise decision when making significant medical decisions.

Professionals may sometimes view denial negatively, expressing frustration at a parent's apparent unwillingness to move more quickly on recommendations following a diagnosis. However, denial is a mechanism that helps protect individuals from emotional pain that they are not yet able to face. Parents need time to adjust to the new reality they are confronting. The amount of time necessary to accept the presence of a disorder varies greatly. Professionals should only become concerned when inaction becomes protracted and threatens to impact negatively on the child. It is also important to recognize that inaction may be a result of other factors such as limited financial resources, lack of family support, feelings of inadequacy, or cultural differences. Listening carefully to caregivers as they talk about their reactions will help to identify what mechanisms are at play. It may be necessary to provide additional support from social workers or other professionals to ease burdens and promote the grieving process.

Resistance

Resistance, the second state common to the grieving process, often overlaps with denial (Luterman, 2001). An individual who is resistant expresses understanding that a disorder is present, but often denies that it will affect the family or the affected member to any significant degree. A caregiver may make comments that wearing the hearing aid is only a temporary situation or insist that wearing the hearing aids will only be necessary while the child is in school. In the case of Waardenburg syndrome, there may be acceptance of the hearing loss in that specific family member, but an unwillingness to accept that it may manifest in other family members. There also may be an unwillingness to share with other family members that Waardenburg is suspected, to have hearing tests done on the whole family, or to have genetic counseling.

Affirmation and Integration

Affirmation and integration are two states that may also blend together to a certain degree. During both affirmation and integration, the presence of the hearing loss (and in WS the presence of the genetic disorder) is openly acknowledged. The primary difference between the two states is the way in which the disorder is viewed. During affirmation, the family may define itself or the family member in terms of the disorder. In affirmation, a parent has a hearing-impaired or deaf child. In contrast, when a disorder is integrated into the life of the family, there is a child who has many characteristics one of which is hearing loss. A family that has integrated the diagnosis of WS will be one that acknowledges its presence and takes appropriate actions such as having genetic counseling and regular hearing tests, but they do not define themselves in terms of the presence of the disorder.

Unresolved Grief

If a caregiver is still actively searching for a cause long after the diagnosis it is possible they have not completed the process of grieving. Additional indicators include depression, inability to deal effectively with emotions, lack of emotion, continuing to seek a different diagnosis, defensiveness, passivity, and confusion (Yoshinago-Itano, 2001). Evidence suggests that age of identification may be related to grief resolution with the parents of older children demonstrating more difficulty in progressing through the grief process. Late identification of hearing loss is often associated with more delayed language development, which is speculated to have an impact on maternal bonding. Caregivers who are having difficulty accepting or coping with the diagnosis of hearing loss in the family should be provided with or referred for counseling.

The progression through grief is often variable. Caregivers may spend more time in one state or return to a state more than once as they work to integrate the diagnosis into the lives of their family. As the child grows older, periodic setbacks such as progression of the hearing loss may result in a return to grief. However, individuals who have successfully worked through the various emotions following the initial diagnosis will be able to move more rapidly through the process when events trigger a renewed sense of loss (Yoshinago-Itano, 2001).

It is interesting to note that, although parents grieve when a child is diagnosed with hearing loss, the emotional experience for the child can be very different. When a hearing loss is identified early, children grow up with the knowledge that they have a hearing loss. Any differences they experience in auditory perception become a part of their everyday lives and therefore normal for them. Some parents understand this intellectually, but emotionally may project their own fear of experiencing hearing loss onto the child. They may also fear their child will be treated differently by others or encounter difficulties in school or later in the workplace. Parental concerns regarding a child's happiness are universal. However, the hearing loss provides a focus for them. In addition, the caregiver often believes that the hearing loss will be an additional burden that a child should not have to bear.

A recent interview with a 15-year-old with a progressive sensorineural hearing loss associated with WS exemplifies the difference in perceptions between mother and son. The mother described her reaction to learning about the hearing loss and working through the emotions in a pattern similar to that previously described. She talked about the shock and later the pain of accepting the presence of the loss and her fears that the hearing loss was getting worse. In contrast, during a private interview, the child stated that the hearing loss was something that he experienced every day and he had no memory of having perfect hearing. Although he understood his mother was concerned about the potential changes in his hearing, he was doing well and was confident of his ability to cope with changes as they occurred.

EMOTIONS ASSOCIATED WITH THE INITIAL DIAGNOSIS AND LONG-TERM ADJUSTMENT

Anger

A number of emotions may arise as part of the process of adjusting to the diagnosis. For example, denial and resistance may be accompanied by anger. Anger can be a powerful defense mechanism, especially when it pertains to a parent's desire to protect their child. The anger can be expressed overtly, such as through accusations that the testing was inadequate or poorly done, or covertly, as when the family leaves and never returns to the office even when the diagnosis has been confirmed by another professional. In the latter instance, the parent associates the pain of the diagnosis with the individual who delivers the news and is unable to bring him- or herself to interact with this person further. The family may also express anger when there are not immediate answers to such questions as "will the hearing loss get worse?" and "will my other children have hearing loss?" The anger in this case is born out of frustration and concern that they do have information and now may need to take further action or of fear that there will be further pain for themselves and their child.

It is easy to become defensive in the face of a patient's anger. We want to make sure patients know we have done the appropriate testing and that we are doing our best to help them find answers. However, answering anger with a barrage of facts is usually ineffective. I recommend that the professional acknowledge the presence of the anger and try to help the patient cope more effectively with it by identifying the associated emotions. Open-ended questions and reflective statements can both be useful. Some examples include; "Tell me more about the anger you are feeling." "It must be very frightening to think about the things we have discussed today." Maintaining a calm demeanor and speaking in a soft voice are also helpful. It is more difficult to maintain anger when the individual to whom you are speaking does not reflect impatience or irritation.

Sadness

Students often report that, next to anger, dealing with a caregiver's or patient's expression of emotional pain is the most intimidating counseling experience. When watching a person cry, it is a natural reaction to want to ease the pain and students want to know the magic words to make the patient (and consequently the student) feel better. Unfortunately, there are no magic words. The most appreciated response a health care professional can provide is quiet support. If the caregiver apologizes for his or her reaction, it is always appropriate to reassure patients that it is all right for them to express themselves. Give them time to recover and privacy if they request it, but do not leave the room as a way to avoid your own discomfort. Your presence is a strong statement of your willingness to help.

Guilt

Luterman (2001) indicates that guilt seems especially prevalent when the condition is congenital. Indicators that there is a genetic syndrome present can be a two-edged sword. Caregivers are often driven by the desire to find out the cause of the hearing loss so they have a place to focus their emotions and to gain a better understanding of the situation. Information can provide a sense of control in a situation where families are feeling a sense of vulnerability. On the other hand, a genetic loss implies that some member of the family is responsible for introducing the "flaw" into the family line. The side of the family or the individual who is suspected of introducing the syndrome can become demonized. The individual who carries the gene can feel tremendous guilt. Although the health care professional can provide facts in an attempt to counteract guilt, facts are often ineffective, especially in the face of the reality that an individual may, in fact, be the carrier of the gene to which the hearing loss is linked. Once again, acknowledging the presence of the guilt is the most effective approach. If persistent guilt seems to be interfering with the individual family's coping effectively with the situation, it is always appropriate to make a referral for counseling. If there are religious undertones to the guilt as illustrated by such statements as "I can't understand why my family would be punished like this," consider making a referral to a faith-based counselor who can approach the issue from within the context of the family's belief system. Such professionals are trained counselors, but provide services from the perspective of particular religious faiths.

Relief

It may surprise some professionals when a caregiver expresses relief following the diagnosis. Some caregivers have been suspicious for some time that their child is "different" from other children in appearance or behavior. Well-meaning health care professionals, friends, or other family members may have dismissed their concerns with statements like "they will out grow it," "she or he is just slow," or "she is a delightful child, relax and enjoy her." The caregiver has had to pursue answers to questions independent of support from those closest to them. When a professional acknowledges that a disorder is present, the caregiver experiences a sense of validation. For the first time, they have found someone who confirms the accuracy of their observations. They are no longer the overly anxious parent or nosy grandparent. Other family members may still resist the diagnosis, but at least someone is there to provide the caregiver with support as he or she tries to make changes that will benefit the child. In addition, a specific diagnosis provides a focus for emotion. The unnamed fear can be more difficult to address.

GENETIC COUNSELING

The complexity of emotions involved may be one reason that some families who appear to have WS (based on physical traits and/or information from the family history) are unwilling to undergo genetic counseling to verify the presence of the gene. Health care professionals need to be prepared for a mixed response to the suggestion that a hearing loss may be the result of WS. Two separate grieving processes come into play. As previously discussed, individuals in the family may ultimately accept the presence of the hearing loss, and openly discuss the possibility of WS with other family members, but resist genetic testing. Family 2, described in chapter 5, is an example of such a case. For several generations the family had viewed their distinctive physical features such as mottled eyes as an identifying family trait that unified them. It is now difficult to fully accept that those features may be associated with deafness. Subject 4 has been trying to alert and educate family members regarding the possibility of WS and has expressed concern for future generations, but she elected not to pursue genetic counseling for herself or her children even when it was made available at no cost. A positive result from the tests would erase any positive connotation for the physical traits prized by the family and confirm the presence of a gene that can create heartache for parents and grandparents. A confirmation of the gene also means that family members will be faced with difficult decisions such as whether to tell potential spouses that the gene is a part of the family history. By avoiding genetic testing, the decisions can also be avoided, as can the process of working through to acceptance of the presence of WS. By not having the test, hope can still exists that WS is not a part of the genetic profile.

In contrast, Family 1, subject 1 was initially hesitant, but following the birth of their first child and at the urging of the wife, they completed genetic counseling. Their stated reason for following through on genetic testing was that they wanted to have the information to prepare for possible hearing loss and to be able to make informed decisions.

Adults with WS

When adults are diagnosed with hearing loss, their reactions may follow the grief stages presented previously. The primary difference is that adults know at some level when they are experiencing difficulty with communication; therefore, they usually do not report feeling shock when the diagnosis of hearing loss is made. Denial, however, is quite common with any type of adult-onset hearing loss. Blame is often placed on others. Wives are accused of speaking with soft voices from other parts of the house and husbands are accused of poor speaking habits. Some individuals may be unwilling to accept the possibility that the loss is genetic and blame noise exposure, early childhood illness, or other health problems. Others may express a keen interest in the possibility as it may provide an explanation for a hearing loss when no other causes can be identified.

For example, one of my patients had a hearing loss beginning at a young age and reported that it had steadily progressed throughout her life. Her parents had associated the loss with childhood illness. After noticing the unusual teal blue color of her eyes, I suggested she return for a more extensive interview and history to include a craniofacial examination. The results suggested that there was a high probability the hearing loss was related to Waardenburg syndrome and genetic testing was recommended. The patient was enthusiastic about the prospect of obtaining more information about the potential cause of her hearing loss. It remains to be seen whether her family will share her interest.

Genetic Counseling and Cultural Diversity

Research on genetic counseling has revealed some interesting differences in attitudes toward prenatal genetic testing for deafness and hard-of-hearing conditions. A survey of 96 normal-hearing parents of children with hearing loss found that 96% of the respondents approved of genetic testing and 87% felt that it should be done parentally (Brunger et al., 2000). In contrast, a survey which included individuals who were deaf, hard of hearing, and normal hearing with parents who were either deaf or children who were deaf revealed some very different attitudes (Middleton, 2004). In addition, the respondents who were deaf represented individuals who considered themselves culturally Deaf (used sign language to communicate and associated more with the Deaf community rather than hearing community) and individuals who considered themselves nonculturally deaf.

When asked if they would have prenatal genetic testing for deafness, 49% of the hearing individuals said "yes," 39% said "no," and 12% responded "not sure." In the hard-of-hearing group, 39% said "yes," 48% said "no," and 13% were "unsure." Twenty-one percent of the deaf respondents indicated they would have prenatal testing, 68% said "no," and 11% were "unsure." When the results were analyzed in terms of individuals who associated with the Deaf culture, 18% were interested in prenatal genetic testing, 76% were not, and 9% were "unsure."

When considering the results of the two studies and the high percentage of positive responses obtained by Brunger et al. (2000), it should be noted that the phrasing of the questionnaires used in the two studies appeared to differ. For example, Middleton (2004) asked: "Would you have a test in pregnancy for deafness?" as compared to statements such as: "Do you believe genetic testing should be offered prenatally?" (Brunger et al., 2000). There is apparently a potentially significant difference in perception between whether testing should be available and whether an individual would choose to have it done for him- or herself or their family members. This is illustrated by the drop of positive responses from an overall 96% positive view of genetic testing to 76% when Brunger et al. asked subjects if they would have genetic testing done on themselves to 72% when asked if they were interested in having their deaf child tested. Of parents who were interested in having the deaf child tested, only 44% were interested in having the other children tested as well. Brunger et al. point out that, in many cases, respondents' perceptions may have been affected by a poor understanding of genetics in general (such as understanding siblings might be carriers) and an underlying fear of how test results might be used. Both studies support the need for guidelines on how to conduct genetic counseling to ensure that families understand the information they have been given, how the results will be handled, and how the family may choose to use them.

The results of these two surveys also serve to illustrate the diversity of opinions on issues related to genetic testing for conditions related to hearing loss. Therefore, when counseling patients about the possibility of seeking genetic counseling, it is important that some attempt is made to explore the patient's attitude toward deafness and toward genetic testing as separate issues. The discussion can then be focused on the positive attributes of genetic testing most appropriate for the individual's belief system. The two studies also provided insights into the different reasons individuals might choose to have genetic testing. Middleton (2004) found the two reasons most often selected by all three participating groups (deaf, hard-of-hearing, and hearing) were to "prepare myself personally for the child's needs" and "prepare for the language needs of my child." A third reason that also was selected often was to "avoid putting my child through unnecessary medical tests." Of the 32 subjects in Brunger et al. study (2000) who had genetic testing on their child, 92% indicated they wanted to know the cause of the hearing loss. Health care professionals are in a position to help families understand that information can be a very powerful tool in helping them cope with the diagnosis of WS and the associated hearing loss.

SPECIAL CONSIDERATIONS WHEN WORKING WITH FAMILIES WITH WS

Families with WS may find themselves feeling "out of the loop" with respect to sources of information and support. Unlike other disorders, there are no highly publicized support groups. The general public is usually unfamiliar with the name or the consequences of WS. Health care professionals can be the means to provide the understanding families are seeking. By making the effort to encourage regular hearing evaluations for the family, professionals can maintain contact and, thereby, provide a sense of continuity and support. Annual evaluations also provide a forum for family members to talk about WS with each other and share new information and connections family members have made during the past year. In the event the family has decided not to pursue genetic counseling to confirm the presence of the gene, the regular gatherings provide a means to track changes in attitude and emotional concerns that may lead to greater acceptance. Asking family members if they are willing to be contacted by other families on your case load and encouraging the different groups to talk to one another about their experiences can also be helpful. The variation in the possible hearing loss configurations, the time of onset, and the potential for the hearing loss to progress create uncertainty that is difficult for individuals from other families to understand. In the absence of formal support groups, knowing that other families with WS have undergone and continue to struggle with the similar issues is often very comforting.

SUMMARY

When counseling families with WS-related hearing loss, the primary goal of the health care professional is to remain flexible in the face of uncertainty. Each family brings to the table different dynamics and personal experiences that will shape their reactions to the hearing loss. The most effective and important skill that the health care professional has is that of empathetic listening. A family in shock will not remember the facts you provided using an impressive list of references with incidence figures and flow charts. They will, however, recall whether you showed compassion, concern, and a willingness to help them work through the mysteries of coping with a hearing loss associated with WS.

REFERENCES

Brunger, J. W., Murray, G. S., O'Riordan, M., Matthews, A. L., Smith, R. J., & Robin, N. H. (2000). Parental attitudes toward genetic testing for pediatric deafness. *American Journal of Human Genetics*, *67*, 1621–1625.

Buckman, R. (1992). *How to break bad news: A guide for health care professionals.* Baltimore, MD: The John Hopkins University Press.

Clark, J., & English, K. (2004). *Counseling in audiology practice*. Boston: Pearson Education Inc.

Kovarsky, D., Kurtzer-White, E., & Maxwell, M. (2004). Stories of origin in the identification of hearing loss among neonates. *Seminars in Hearing*, *25*, 319–332.

Kubler-Ross, E. (1969). *On death and dying*. New York: Macmillan Publishing Co.

Luterman, D. (2001). *Counseling persons with communication disorders and their families*. Austin, TX: Pro-Ed.

Middleton, A. (2004). Deaf and hearing adult's attitudes toward genetic testing for deafness (pp.127–147). In J. V. Van Cleve (Ed.), *Genetics and disability, and deafness*. Washington, DC: Gallaudet University Press.

Rogers, C. (1951) *Patient centered therapy*. Boston: Houghton Mifflin.

Skotko, B. (2005a). Mothers of children with Down syndrome reflect on their postnatal support. *Pediatrics*, *115*, 64–77.

Skotko, B. (2005b). Postnatal support of mothers of children with Down syndrome. *Mental Retardation*, *43*, 196–212.

Yoshinago-Itano, C. (2001) The social emotional ramifications of universal newborn hearing screening, early identification and intervention of children who are deaf and hard of hearing. In R. Seewald. & J. Gravel (Eds.), *A sound foundation through early amplification: Proceedings of the second international conference* (pp. 221–231). Edmundsbury, UK: St. Edmundsbury Press.

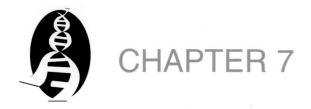

CHAPTER 7

Treatment Issues for Patients with Waardenburg Syndrome

*C*hapters 4, 5, and 6 presented plans for differential diagnosis of WS, for diagnosing and treating hearing loss resulting from WS, and for counseling families who have WS-related hearing losses. Diagnosis of WS is usually followed by referrals to the specialists who are most capable of treating the effects of WS: an audiologist, speech-language pathologist, genetic counselor, or, when appropriate, a craniofacial team. Appropriate referrals are no guarantee that patients will comply with the recommendations or attend appropriate therapy. Even patients who are receiving therapy may still have unresolved issues about WS. This chapter summarizes some of the treatment issues that may facilitate or hinder a patient's successful recovery from the effects of WS and includes suggestions for recognizing and dealing with impediments to treatment plans. After reading this chapter you will be able to:

■ List four reasons that patients may refuse or reject diagnostic outcomes and treatment recommendations regarding WS.

■ Compare several organizations that provide professional assistance in diagnosing and treating WS.

■ List several support organizations that can assist patients with WS to overcome the problems associated with WS.

■ List two professional organizations that can help health care professionals solve WS-related treatment problems.

PATIENTS' REACTIONS TO TREATMENT PLANS

Patients with WS are individuals with unique needs. In previous chapters, we learned the most common problems associated with WS and how those problems are diagnosed. We also reviewed some options for treating the effects of WS. Patients may react in several ways to treatment plans: they may choose to ignore their problems and hope they will resolve themselves (reject the plan of treatment); they may defer following the treatment plan until they are able to accept the diagnosis and move on toward resolution; or they may begin the appropriate therapy to overcome the effects of WS immediately.

FACTORS AFFECTING TREATMENT OF WS

Suppose, even after obtaining evidence that WS is the cause of the patient's problem, the patient or the patient's family decides not to follow the recommendations for seeking genetic assessment and/or genetic counseling. What should the health care professional do in such cases?

No matter how patients react regarding treatment recommendations, they and their families need the continued support, understanding, and patience of the health care professionals who referred them for treatment. Chapter 6 discussed the need of patients to complete a grieving process before they are able to take appropriate action to deal with a hearing loss. Unresolved emotions about the implications of a genetic disorder are certainly a factor in a patient's reaction to treatment plans for WS. Other factors are at work as well, including lack of information regarding the treatment plans, financial concerns, and emotional and psychological support for the entire family. Health care professionals are capable of easing these concerns through patient education, appropriate contact with other professionals, and continued contact with the families of patients with WS.

Patient Education

Patients may harbor misconceptions about some of the recommendations, particularly the recommendation that the family seek genetic counseling. Some families may resist genetic counseling for a variety of reasons, including perceptions about expense, privacy issues, or religious beliefs regarding birth control and therapeutic abortion (see shaded box on following page).

Myths About Genetic Counseling

- **MYTH:** A genetic counselor will tell me not to have children.
- **TRUTH:** Reputable genetic counselors predict the odds of having offspring with particular conditions. For example, if one parent has the autosomal dominant form of WS1, and the other parent does not have the gene for this condition, the probability of a child being born with WS1 is 50%, or 1 out of 2 children. Reputable genetic counselors never advise individuals to refrain from having children. Genetic counselors predict the odds of occurrence of specific genetic events based on family pedigrees, and phenotypic and genotypic test results. It is up to the family to decide whether or not the risk factors of having a child with a genetic condition outweigh the possibility of having a "normal" child.

- **MYTH:** If a genetic counselor finds a genetic problem he or she will advise me to terminate my pregnancy.
- **TRUTH:** Genetic counselors present patients with an array of possibilities. For example, if genetic analysis indicates that a pregnant woman has a fetus with Down syndrome, the woman has several choices. She may decide to have the baby and place it for adoption; she may decide to have the baby and raise it at home; she may decide to terminate the pregnancy and adopt a "normal" child; she may decide to terminate the pregnancy and try to become pregnant with a "normal" child some time in the future. Although there are prenatal tests for some forms of the WS gene, there are currently no prenatal tests for WS-related hearing loss, cleft palate, and Hirschsprung's megacolon. These conditions cannot presently be detected by genetic testing. This means that, although the gene for WS may be detected prenatally, the highly variable phenotypic effects of the gene cannot. Prenatal counseling on options for diagnosing and treating hearing loss are desirable if there is a strong family history of deafness. In all cases, the parents, not the genetic counselor, make the decisions about childbearing.

- **MYTH:** I know the baby I am carrying is not my husband's child. If I go to a genetic counselor she will discover this and tell my husband.
- **TRUTH:** This myth has some truth. A genetic counselor may in fact discover that the child cannot be the biological child of the legal father. However, the counselor must respect the patient's privacy and wishes, and will not ethically reveal this finding

without the mother's permission. There is a possibility for legal action and paternity testing in the future, depending on the state of the marriage, but that is an issue apart from genetic testing to determine the presence or cause of a genetic syndrome.

- **MYTH:** Genetic testing and genetic counseling will determine the cause of my problems with 100% accuracy
- **TRUTH:** No medical test is 100% accurate, including genetic tests. Genetic testing has yet to be developed or perfected for many syndromes, including WS types 2B, 2C, and 2D, as well as WS2 with ocular albinism.

- **MYTH:** My religious beliefs prevent me from using birth control or having an abortion. There is no reason to have genetic testing or counseling because I won't do anything to stop a pregnancy anyway.
- **TRUTH:** There are other benefits of genetic testing and counseling besides preventing the birth of a child with a syndrome. In the case of WS, the family may decide to have children even at the risk of having a deaf child. Counselors can help family members prepare for postnatal detection and treatment of hearing loss in the newborn child. The family may want to know the options for treatment of a hard-of-hearing child, including choice of communication system, possibility of cochlear implantation, hearing aid selection, and educational opportunities for children with hearing loss.

- **MYTH:** Genetic counseling isn't worth the expense.
- **TRUTH:** Genetic counseling is an expensive investment. However, this investment pays off by helping the family make decisions and plans that may reduce expenses long-term. Genetic counselors sometimes know of research programs that offer free diagnostics and low-cost or free treatment. At the very least, they can help the family estimate the long-term expenses involved in rearing a child with WS, and predict the odds of having more children with WS.

As health care professionals we are accustomed to treating serious medical conditions, including those of genetic etiology. Our familiarity with serious conditions sometimes makes us forget how frightening and unacceptable these conditions may seem to individuals who are experiencing these problems for the first time. Although we hope the family will immediately seek treatment and counseling, it seldom works this way. The news that a genetic problem may be the cause of a medical condition is often met with feelings of guilt, denial, and fear. These fears may be coupled with misunderstandings about genetic issues in general. Specific financial and social concerns may also hinder treatment. Here are some things to keep in mind while discussing treatment options with the family:

- Give the family time to adjust to the news that the problem has a genetic basis. Adjustment time varies from several months to several years. A few individuals refuse to ever accept the diagnosis and either "doctor shop" for additional diagnoses or ignore the problem altogether. Most families, in my experience, fall somewhere in between immediate acceptance and complete denial of a condition.

- Offer the family the opportunity to meet and talk with individuals who have identical or similar problems. I have several families of patients with WS who welcome the opportunity to counsel and educate other patients who have WS. Seeing how others have successfully handled the problems associated with WS is often enough incentive to get new patients to begin long-range planning, including genetic counseling. If WS support personnel are not available locally, suggest that the family contact the WS support Web site (http://www.muohio.edu/waardenburgsyndrome/). This site offers family members the opportunity to interact with individuals who have WS or with parents who have children with WS.

- Realize that the family may have reasons for avoiding counseling and may have family information that they have not revealed to you. This information is not always related to genetic issues, although sometimes it is. Patients may be in this country illegally, may be using controlled substances recreationally, may fear they have AIDS or a sexually transmitted disease, may be wanted for criminal misconduct, or may be the subject of paternity disputes. They may correctly fear that blood work will reveal health issues that they may wish to keep secret.

- Realize that one or both of the "parents" of the proband may not actually be the biological parents of the child. Situations may arise in which the mother of a child may refuse genetic counseling because she fears that the real paternity of the child may be exposed to the child's "father." This situation may arise when the child is the product of incest, rape, or an extramarital affair.

- Understand that religious or ethnic beliefs may affect how the family responds to WS. The family may believe that genetic counseling or family planning violates "accepting God's will" for the birth of children, for example.

- Continue to find opportunities to educate the family about WS. The more the family members understand the condition, the more likely they are to take steps to resolve it.

■ Treat the *effects* of the syndrome whether or not the family decides to seek genetic counseling. Examples of the effects of WS include language delay, and resonance, voice, and articulation issues if cleft palate is part of the phenotype. Hearing loss is always a possibility in patients with WS, and aggressive diagnostic and treatment plans are warranted for persons with this syndrome. Surgery may be required for cleft palate, aganglionic megacolon, or for cosmetic reasons to improve facial appearance. Keep the family a part of the treatment planning process, and inform them of progress, and of the long-term outlook for the treatment procedures.

■ Realize that for members of the Deaf community, deafness is regarded as normal. Deaf parents may welcome the possibility of having a Deaf child as a desirable option. Do not assume that information about hearing loss is unwelcome.

■ Periodically reintroduce the idea of genetic counseling as a desirable option for family treatment. Families often do change their thinking after they adjust to the idea of a genetic cause for their medical problem.

RESOURCES FOR REFERRAL AND TREATMENT OF PATIENTS WITH WS

Some health care professionals work in medical centers with multiple resources for referral and treatment within their facility. However, professionals who are not equipped to diagnose and treat rare or uncommon syndromes must rely on outside resources to help formulate the best plan of care for patients with WS. Several resources are available for professionals who need help treating patients with syndromes in general, and WS in particular.

American Cleft Palate Craniofacial Association (ACPA)

The ACPA is an international, multidisciplinary medical society composed of members who treat patients with anomalies of the head and face. In addition to publishing the previously described team directory, the ACPA also publishes the bimonthly *Cleft Palate-Craniofacial Journal*. This journal is available in print, or online to ACPA members, or in medical libraries. Membership in the ACPA provides access to a list serve that is an extremely valuable resource for those of us who work with patients who have syndromes or craniofacial anomalies. ACPA membership is open to health care professionals. For information on current membership dues and benefits visit the Web site at http://www.acpa-cpf.org/. The ACPA also publishes informational pamphlets for patient education purposes, and a portion of the Web site is open to the public to provide answers about cleft lip, cleft palate, and syndromes affecting the head and face.

American Speech-Language-Hearing Association (ASHA)

The American Speech-Language-Hearing Association is the certifying body for speech-language pathologists (SLPs) and audiologists. ASHA membership provides SLPs and audiologists with a wide variety of continuing education opportunities, including workshops and conventions with presentations on genetics and hearing loss. It publishes five professional journals, that are available on-line to members, and offers 16 Special Interest Divisions for specific professional interests. Visit the Web site at http://www.asha.org to learn more about continuing education opportunities in the areas of genetics and hearing loss.

Genetic/Rare Conditions Support Groups

Health care professionals who need information about rare genetic conditions can access this information at http://www.kumc.edu/gec/support. This Web site was developed by the University of Kansas Medical Center and helps health care professionals locate genetic counselors, government consumer health information, and national and international support organizations for individuals with genetic conditions. It is open to the general public, as well as to professionals interested in genetic problems.

Online Mendelian Inheritance in Man (OMIM)

Dr. Victor McKusick and colleagues developed this database catalog of genetic disorders at Johns Hopkins. It is designed for use by physicians and geneticists, and for persons who want advanced scientific information on specific genetic disorders. The Web site is available at http://www.3.ncbi.nlm.nih.gov/omim/.

RESOURCES FOR INDIVIDUALS WITH WS

About Face

Patients who have facial anomalies often benefit from interacting with other people who have similar anomalies. About Face is a support organization for patients who have congenital or acquired facial anomalies. It is also a useful resource for professionals who work with such patients. The organization's Web site is http://www.aboutfaceusa.org/.

Girls and Boys Town

The Girls and Boys Town organization has a research registry for hereditary hearing loss. The site collects information from families and individuals who wish to participate in hearing loss-related research. In addition to providing information about WS and other genetic syndromes, the site also has links to current research projects and surveys about hereditary hearing loss. See http://www.girlsandboystown.org/ for more information about hereditary hearing loss in general, and WS in particular, or e-mail them at deafgenereg istry@boystown.org.

Gallaudet University

Gallaudet University in Washington D.C. has long been known for its excellent educational programs for deaf individuals. In addition to deaf education, the faculty and support staff also provide a genetics program for the Deaf community. This program has studied the ethical implications of genetic testing for deafness, and provides genetic evaluation and counseling as well as genetic testing to individuals with hereditary hearing loss (Arnos & Pandya, 2004).

Gallaudet also has an excellent genetics training program each summer for audiologists who want to learn more about genetic forms of deafness. To learn more about Gallaudet and continuing education offerings for health care professionals, access their Web site at http://www.gallaudet.edu.

Other Organizations

Several other organizations provide information on deafness in general, and WS in particular. These include:

American Society for Deaf Children
P.O. Box 3355
Gettysburg, PA 17325
Phone: 800-942-2732 (parent hotline);
717-334-7922 (business V/TTY)
Fax: 717-334-8808
E-mail: asdc@deafchildren.org
Web site: http://www.deafchildren.org

Hereditary Hearing Loss Home Page
http://www.webhost.us.ac.be/hhh

National Association of the Deaf
814 Thayer Avenue
Silver Spring, MD 20910

Phone: 301-587-1788 (voice); 301-587-1789 (TTY)
Fax: 301-587-1791
E-mail: NADinfo@nad.org
Web site: http://www.nad.org

WS SUPPORT GROUPS

Because we were unable to locate national WS support groups or Web sites devoted only to WS, we at Miami University of Ohio have developed a support group and Web site. The Web site, http://www.muohio.edu/waardenburg syndrome/, contains updated contact information, details experiences of individuals with WS, and provides descriptions and photographs of anomalies associated with WS. If you are an individual with WS, a family member related to someone who has WS, or a professional whose patients may be interested in joining a support group, please contact us through the Web site or in one of the following ways:

- E-mail: Kahna@muohio.edu

- Regular mail: Alice Kahn, Ph.D., Dept. of Speech Pathology and Audiology, 2 Bachelor Hall, Miami University, Oxford, OH 45056, USA

- FAX: 513-529-2502

- Telephone with voice mail: 513-529-2508

FUTURE DIRECTIONS

Current information about WS leaves much to be desired. Better methods of diagnosis and treatment of WS are still evolving. Locations and effects of the WS genes are under investigation, as are the phenotypic features and treatment options for patients with WS-related problems. Some preliminary studies have offered hope that one day, not only the genes for all types of WS, but the phenotypic effects of the genes will be identified through prenatal testing. In the meantime, we as health care professionals can do our part by:

- Recognizing the phenotypic signs of WS in our patients

- Recommending appropriate audiologic testing of infants born at risk for WS

- Diagnosing and treating hearing loss in patients with WS

■ Referring patients with multiple physical problems to craniofacial teams for long-term planning and treatment

■ Recommending genetic counseling for families with WS

■ Recommending psychological counseling for patients who have unresolved emotional issues regarding WS

■ Treating the effects of WS: articulation disorders, cleft palate, spina bifida, Hirschsprung's megacolon, language delay, and hearing loss

■ Assisting our patients to locate diagnostic, educational, and support resources

■ Educating ourselves on the latest WS genetic and audiologic research.

Laboratories Providing Clinical Testing of WS

Several genetic laboratories offer clinical testing for WS. Remember that clinical testing is not yet available for all types of WS, and that not every lab provides all types of available tests.

■ Boston University School of Medicine
Center for Human Genetics, Boston, MA
Aubrey Milunsky, M.D., D.Sc.

This lab offers genetic sequencing and prenatal diagnosis of WS 1 and WS 2A

■ Chapman Institute/Center for Genetic Testing at St. Francis
Genetics Laboratory, Tulsa, OK
Nancy Carpenter, Ph.D., F.A.C.M.G.;
Frederick V. Schaefer, Ph.D., F.A.C.M.G.

Lab provides genetic sequencing and prenatal diagnosis of WS 1, WS 2A, and WS 3

■ University of Nebraska Medical Center
Human Genetics Laboratory, Munroe-Meyer Institute
Omaha, NE
Warren G. Sanger, Ph.D.

Lab provides FISH-metaphase and FISH-Interphase for WS1 and WS3
Also provides genetic sequencing and prenatal diagnosis of WS2A

Most of all, we can be aware of the possibility that genetic factors may be the cause of some or all of the problems of the patients we are treating. Treating those problems and sharing our results is one step all of us can take toward a universal resolution of the problems facing WS patients everywhere.

REFERENCE

Arnos, K. S., & Panday, A. (2004). Genes for deafness and the genetics program at Gallaudet University. In: J. V. Van Cleve (Ed.), *Genetics, disability, and deafness* (pp. 111–126). Washington, DC: Gallaudet University Press.

Index